A KISS THROUGH GLASS

A KISS THROUGH GLASS

Shirley Nolan's
inspirational story
has saved thousands
of lives and offers
hope for the
future

Foreword by
Henny Braund MBE
Preface by Professor
Alejandro Madrigal OBE

SHIRLEY NOLAN

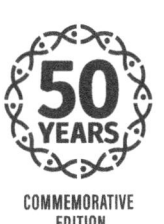

COMMEMORATIVE
EDITION

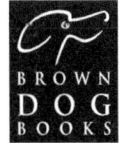

First published in 1978
This edition published in 2024

Copyright © Shirley Nolan 1978, 2024

The right of Shirley Nolan to be identified as the author of this work has been asserted in accordance with the Copyright, Designs & Patents Act 1988.

All rights reserved. No part of this book may be reproduced, stored in a retrieval system, or transmitted in any form or by any means, digital, electronic, electrostatic, magnetic tape, mechanical, photocopying, recording or otherwise, without the written permission of the copyright holder.

Published under licence by Brown Dog Books and The Self-Publishing Partnership Ltd, 10b Greenway Farm, Bath Rd, Wick, nr. Bath BS30 5RL, UK

www.selfpublishingpartnership.co.uk

ISBN printed book: 978-1-83952-808-8
Cover design by Kevin Rylands
Internal design by Mac Style

Printed and bound in the UK

This book is printed on FSC® certified paper

Dedicated to Dr David James of Westminster Hospital, London, for his vision, courage and personal achievement and to my mother, Rhoda Oakey, for her constant love and devotion to Anthony.

– Shirley Nolan

Contents

Foreword	ix
Preface	xii
Patients, Donors, and Supporters	xv
Book One	1
Chapter 1	3
Chapter 2	12
Chapter 3	17
Chapter 4	20
Chapter 5	26
Chapter 6	35
Chapter 7	49
Chapter 8	66
Chapter 9	79
Book Two	95
Chapter 10	97
Chapter 11	109

Chapter 12	119
Chapter 13	131
Chapter 14	141
Chapter 15	156
Chapter 16	167
Chapter 17	174
Chapter 18	180
Chapter 19	121
Chapter 20	199
Chapter 21	204
Epilogue	215

Foreword

There is some purpose behind it all, isn't there?
– Shirley Nolan

In 1974 Shirley Nolan created the world's first register of bone marrow donors. As she searched for a donor for her desperately ill son, Anthony, she couldn't believe there wasn't a panel of potential donors for patients with life-threatening blood disorders or blood cancer. Up until the 1970s, bone marrow transplants from unrelated donors had been singularly unsuccessful. The medical establishment had rejected the treatment as a dead end. But while living in Australia, Shirley had heard about a successful transplant in a London hospital. This was the news that sparked her into action, shaping the course of her life and our history.

This book is a deeply personal and powerful account. Those who have cared for a loved one with a life-threatening illness will recognise the rollercoaster of emotions she describes, from guilt, anguish, and self-doubt to joy in small things, as well as the burning determination that drove her onwards. Progress was slow. Twelve years after Shirley set up the Anthony Nolan register, just one patient a month was receiving a transplant in the UK and survival rates were still very low. Against this backdrop, to build a register of donors and challenge clinical practice took guts and determination.

But Shirley was a determined campaigner, driven by the injustice she felt for the children she got to know in hospital whose lives were cruelly stolen from them at a young age. She was inspired by Anthony's courage and his determination to live, against the odds. For her, the struggle to save Anthony's life became a symbol for the rights of the individual in society, where only the powerful appeared to have a voice. The reality of 1970s Britain didn't deter her – from battling NHS funding cuts to long waiting lists, and the added struggle a recession brings while caring for a sick child. The echoes of some of these battles have all too loud a resonance today. Above all, this is the story of a mother. A mother determined to do all she could to save her son. While Shirley's extraordinary passion was documented through the national and international media, her book documents her vulnerability, how inside she felt nothing like the battling super mum of her public image. And even when she lost that fight, when Anthony tragically died at the age of seven, she succeeded in creating the world's first register. Thanks to Shirley, we now give four people a second chance of life every day and 26,500 people across the world have benefited from a bone marrow or stem cell transplant. Anthony did not die in vain.

But there is still so much more to do. Innovation has driven the charity she founded from the very start. Shirley could not have foreseen the advances in cell and gene therapies in recent years, but she would have embraced their potential to give more patients hope that better, kinder, and more effective treatments will become available. We are under no illusions about the enormous responsibility we bear to patients and their loved ones. We keep growing the register, or some patients won't find their match. We tackle the barriers to accessing treatment, or we lose people. We unlock new treatments, or we miss the opportunity to save more lives.

So, we are now focused on three things. We want to make sure every transplant patient not only survives, but also thrives. They can live long and healthy lives with their families. Secondly, everyone must be able to access the treatment and care they need, no matter their background or circumstances. And finally, we want a future where every patient can benefit from our continued research and discovery, to keep pushing the boundaries of what is possible in treatments and cures. We want a future where the cure doesn't make you sicker than the illness itself. A future where a diagnosis is the beginning of *recovery*, not the beginning of the end. A future where every patient who needs us can survive and thrive.

Let's remember the mother who was inspired to think differently to try and save her son. Inspired to be there for the patients of tomorrow – as we are. While celebrating all that has been achieved, let's look to an exciting future. A future full of hope.

Henny Braund MBE
Anthony Nolan Chief Executive Officer

Preface

From the moment I first read about Shirley Nolan's crusade, I was captivated. Her story inspired me to join Anthony Nolan, to create the charity's Research Institute and to spend more than 25 years as its Scientific Director. Although I never had the opportunity to meet her, I have felt very close to Shirley Nolan throughout my life. Her determination to save her son, and to give patients like Anthony the hope of a potential cure, has driven my life's work.

In 1969, Shirley took on the first big challenge and travelled over land to Australia with the man who became her partner, Ted. When they finally arrived, the thing she desired above all was to have a child and Anthony was born in 1971. But he was born with a serious blood disorder, Wiskott Aldrich Syndrome, which threatened to kill him. In her book, Shirley tells of Anthony's suffering and of her distress at learning that he was unlikely to survive beyond the age of two. She writes about how she wanted to run away, how she would rather face death for both her and for Anthony than continue with this struggle.

The miracle came two years later, on Good Friday in 1973. Her neighbour told her about a boy with a similar condition to Anthony who had been transplanted with bone marrow from an unrelated donor in the UK. From there on, nothing was going to stop her. She wrote to the patient's family, to the hospital, and travelled with Anthony to England to find a donor. She secured the doctors' agreement to repeat the risky treatment if a donor could be found. When she reached a dead end in her search, she redoubled her efforts. She invited journalists, cameras and the world's media to interview her in the hope this could help save her son. As she became a well-known campaigner, she started to receive letters and donations from people around the world, from celebrities to those who gave pennies to support her cause. She wrote back to them all.

She channelled all her talents into pursuing her vision, taking her message to anyone who would listen, and showing a ferocious determination to shake-up those who would not. This took immense bravery, and it took guts. It's testament to the justness of her cause that, at Anthony's funeral, a guard of honour was formed by the same policemen who had arrested Shirley in her early campaigning days. And testament to her powers of persuasion that so many of those police officers went on to join the register.

It was Shirley's dream to establish donor registers, not just in the UK but across the world. Her incredible legacy lives on in the 41 million people now registered as potential donors across more than 50 countries. Over the last 50 years, the scientific community both here in the UK and around the world has pushed the boundaries of knowledge. We now know so much more about genetics and the immune system, and the many factors that influence the outcome of a transplant. This scientific discovery means more patients than ever are receiving a transplant. And more patients have the second chance of life that Anthony, tragically, was denied.

The pace of discovery and progress hasn't slowed. Researchers are discovering, developing and trialling new cell and gene therapies that have the potential to transform clinical practice and outcomes for patients. The progress made since 1974 means if Anthony had been born today, he might be treated using a novel cell therapy and research scientists at Anthony Nolan believe he would have a 93% chance of finding a well-matched unrelated donor. This is a dizzying thought – poignantly sad and hopeful in equal measure. The opportunity to make huge strides for patients today and in the next 50 years is enormous. I am honoured to have this opportunity to remember Shirley, to have served in her shadow and to share her story with a new generation, through this remarkable book.

Professor Alejandro Madrigal OBE
Professor of Haematology at University College London

Professor Alejandro Madrigal OBE was appointed as Anthony Nolan's first Scientific Director in 1995 and created the Anthony Nolan Research Institute. Today the Institute has a global reputation for innovation and discovering the impact of HLA matching on stem cell transplant success. Professor Madrigal's contributions to the field of stem cell transplantation have resulted in the lives of countless patients in the UK and worldwide being saved.

Patients, Donors, and Supporters

Shirley Nolan never gave up on her vision to create the world's first stem cell register to find a match for her son, Anthony, and others in need of a lifesaving transplant. The charity she founded in his name helped find a donor for a dear friend of mine and that inspired me to do all I can to help in return.
– Olivia Colman, Patron, Anthony Nolan

I read Shirley's book when I was a teen and always said I would become donor once I was old enough. Little did I know that my relationship with Anthony Nolan would take a different route. Anthony Nolan saved my life, and I couldn't be more grateful.
– Donna, who had a stem cell transplant for aplastic anaemia

Like Anthony, my son Daniel was born with Wiskott-Aldrich syndrome and needed a stem cell transplant to survive. Anthony never found his match, and he died from this illness without a chance. Shirley tried with all her might, and never wanted another person to go through this. And because of this incredible boy and his mummy, our baby was given the chance of life. After months of searching, they told us they'd found a donor for Daniel. We will be forever grateful to Anthony and Shirley for being the reason Daniel is here today.
– Georgie, whose son Daniel who had two stem cell transplants aged one and three

I want to show people the difference a transplant can make and tell them: I'm here because someone once saved my life, you can do that for someone else. Now I work in stem cell research, an exciting area of science that will hopefully help lots of people. We all have the power to help others. Anthony and Shirley's legacy is one amazing example of that.

– Sonal, who had a stem cell transplant as a child

When I was 9 years old, I saw Anthony and Shirley on TV. That was in 1976 and my grandad had died a few years earlier from leukaemia. He was my knight in shining armour, and I was devastated. My mum explained that her cousin aged 12 was also taken by this disease and Anthony had something similar, but a bone marrow transplant could save him. In my child's mind that was easy: I would give him my bone marrow! So, I contacted my local paper who sent my letter to his mum. Shirley wrote back and asked if she could call me. We arranged a date and she kindly explained that I was too young and the issues around compatibility. However, she said they needed funding for research, so I did a sponsored swim to raise money and awareness for Anthony. I was devastated when he died. Anthony effected my life greatly and I have continued to raise money and awareness throughout my life. I was on the register but am too old now, so my children have taken up the baton and registered. Shirley was a brave and inspirational lady who, with her mum, cared for Anthony and gave him the best life she could. Anthony, you are forever in my heart.

– Lisa, Anthony Nolan supporter

Because of them I get to see my children growing up. I get really emotional about it. Without the transplant I probably wouldn't be here. I still have so much to do, so much to give.

– Bianca, who had a stem cell transplant for aplastic anaemia

My donation experience was life-changing, not just for the patient but for myself. The feeling that I got from giving was priceless. At the very core of human nature there's something about helping out others, and that's how donating felt to me. Donating gives hope.
– Femi, stem cell donor

Our daughter Zara didn't have a donor match in the whole world. We are just so glad that Anthony Nolan found her a cord blood match. I can't even imagine how it would feel when you can't find any match. Like Shirley and Anthony, some families still experience that feeling. That's why Anthony Nolan's work is so important. One day we will be able to save every child who needs a transplant.
– Taruna, whose daughter Zara who had a cord blood transplant aged nine

The impact that the transplant has had, it's just the most amazing thing ever. It was hope. That's what I always say to people about Anthony Nolan – they give you hope, when nobody else can. That's why we continue to support Anthony Nolan, so other people get that hope. Without Anthony Nolan, we would not be here as a family. End of story.
– Noreen, whose daughter Ayesha had a stem cell transplant aged 11

My family and I are deeply grateful to Anthony Nolan and to the incredibly generous human being that was willing to donate his cells, and to give me another chance. My donor came from the US, and I found it fascinating to see the level of coordination involved in getting cells from donor to the patient, across the ocean! It has been really touching to see the level of dedication and generosity that goes into getting a stem cell transplant to a patient. Anthony Nolan made it happen for me. They gave me the possibility of a future, and they keep doing this every day with many other

patients – through stem cell transplants but also through research and enabling the development of new cell therapies. I find that admirable and that is why I support their amazing work.
— Jesús, who had a stem cell transplant for acute lymphoblastic leukaemia

Book One

Chapter 1

Through a blur of tears the blood drops spread like poppies, the drip drip synchronising with the tiny heartbeat, down the long glistening tube into my baby. *ENOUGH!* My silent scream reverberated in my head. But the reality of the screams from the metal cot shattered the stillness of the tiny isolation cubicle. I stared at yet another shaven patch on my son's head, at the stark needle inserted there, at the scrap of humanity writhing to free his hands tied to the cot bars to prevent him lacerating his skin, raw with eczema. Ssshhh! Hush, my lamb. Sleep, little baby, sleep, I sang, trying to quell the quavering in my voice to cover my anguish, to ease his.

How well a mother comes to know her baby's cry. Yet on an evening six months previously, when those same screams disturbed me from the nursery in the maternity hospital, I did not then know it was my baby in the agony of a brain haemorrhage. There were three new mums in our room in the Memorial Hospital, North Adelaide, our babies born in the early hours of December 2, 1971. Two of us had nine-pound boys and difficult deliveries and were sedated at night to help us rest. The screams went on and on as I drifted fitfully to sleep.

The nightlight clicked and the glare silhouetted the figures at the foot of the bed. I didn't have to listen. I knew what they were saying. I held up my hands as if that alone could stem the flow of words, but the voices wound on, strangely distorted like a tape slowed down, the moving lips appearing detached from their faces.

No, my God, no! It was my nightmare become reality, like the rescreening of a scene from a play that I had written. My gynaecologist was accompanied by a paediatrician. 'Your baby has sustained a severe brain haemorrhage,' he said. 'He has already been transferred to the Children's Hospital. There is little hope. We're very sorry.' Sorry, I thought. Sorry? My God, I prayed to you every night of my pregnancy for my unborn child. Why? Why? Leave him alone, I shouted. Not, how is he or how did it happen? I knew, didn't I? Leave him alone, I repeated.

I turned my face to the wall. The kind night sister came and held my hands, quietly asking, 'What do you wish him to be christened, my dear?' 'Anthony,' I could barely whisper.

Anthony, I thought. My son. I've held you only for a few minutes. I've tried to give you life, but soon you will be dead. I crushed my face into the pillows and muffled the deep sobs, trying not to disturb my two new friends. But they had heard all and were quietly weeping with me.

My husband Ted and my mother arrived, shocked and upset, trying to offer words of comfort. Mother was ashen and only concerned to comfort me, but I just wanted to be alone. So they left to be with Anthony. A quick injection and the night began to close in about me, pressing me deeper, deeper into the world behind the face. Leave him alone ... leave him alone, was all I remembered saying as I slid into the levels of the past.

* * *

'Why hasn't something happened yet?' I asked Ted as I picked him up from work. My hands were gripping the steering wheel so tightly they left painful crescent indentations in my palms. 'Our baby's at least two weeks overdue. There's something wrong, I just know there is,' I said, becoming more agitated. 'What if he has a brain haemorrhage?' 'Why do you say that?' Ted asked. 'I just sense it, as if I can see what's going to happen,' I cried. 'Now, now, calm down,' he said. 'It won't do you any good to get upset. You have your gynaecologist's appointment tomorrow – I'm sure he'll decide then ... he really can't leave it any longer, can he, or you'll burst.' Ted was trying so hard to be reassuring but I wasn't listening anymore.

I knew the route well through the beautiful parklands to North Adelaide, but my thoughts were in another city. We formerly ran a small freight business from the air terminal in Darwin and after I had stopped work due to my pregnancy I would accompany Ted on his deliveries. We easily filled our days with excited talk of our planned journey soon from Darwin to Adelaide, the house we would build to make a home for the baby, and if it was going to be a boy or a girl. I recall vividly the day we took a crate of therapy equipment to a school for severely mentally and physically handicapped children. The different ones in their twilight world, the staring eyes, grimacing or drooling faces, huge lolling heads, distorted bodies, frenzied jerkings, the limbless and the ones so still like the little fellow sitting beside the gushing tap, his palms outstretched, feeling streams of water between his fingers, his expressionless face raised to the sun and his empty eyes reflecting the tropical sky. I experienced conflicting emotions of heartache, revulsion, pity and fear as the truck rumbled on to Bagot Road and I placed my hands on my rounded growing child within me. But that was in Darwin and it now seemed ages ago.

When I again picked Ted up from work in Adelaide nothing had happened. I had spent the day doing housework, washing the car, shopping, and trudging up and down the flights of steps to our top floor flat, hoping that lots of activity would do the trick. It didn't and the gynaecologist at last agreed to admit me the next day. No dramatic midnight rush for me. It was with resignation and deep foreboding that I entered my assigned room, paced around its strangeness and registered it as mine by planking my toothbrush and toothpaste in the glass above the washbasin. 'Don't worry, love, it will all work out okay,' Ted said but his strained face belied his words. He had to leave shortly afterwards because, of all nights, he had an audition for TV (Ted was a talented singer). Alone, I lay uncomfortable in the hugeness of late pregnancy. I peeled back the crisp sheet, raised my nightie and stroked my tummy, rounded as a ripe pomegranate, and ran my finger round the flattened navel like a miniature whirlpool as if I could see through the spiral, through the stretched skin to the sleeping child within.

Come on little fellow, wake up, get a move on, we've waited a long time for you, I crooned to my unborn. Only the dim reading light focused on my bed like moonlight, leaving the rest of the room swathed in pockets of shadows. In the distance was the faint drone of the city traffic and from the parklands the crickets called. Outside my room at intervals I heard the buzz of voices and accompanying footsteps approach and recede, the clunk and the rumble of trolleys or stretchers, lift doors clanging and, in the distance, intermittent screams. I wondered who was giving life at that exact moment. Here and all over the world, a mammoth birthing was in process. A staggering realisation. I also wondered if other mothers spoke to their babies nestled safely inside them; if, in other lonely little rooms along the corridor, they were doing just this and experiencing the same mixed emotions. But most of all I was wishing to get it all over with. These last weeks of pregnancy seemed so long, especially when according to my calculations I was 20 days overdue. I didn't really know what to expect, despite the books I'd read, the films I'd seen and my keen interest in the experiences related by friends qualified to proffer opinions after their second or third child.

I had a strange feeling that I could just scoop out my baby, divide us as simply as an amoeba. I desperately wanted my baby out of me. Yes, I was afraid. I began praying that I wouldn't die, but most of all that the baby would be healthy and normal. I was overwhelmingly afraid of the actual birth. Not the pain so much as the giving of life, the immense responsibility of growing another person inside of me, yet not knowing who or what was there until the moment of birth. I had experienced this fear for as long as I had been a woman. A recurring premonition? I pulled the sheet up under my chin and slowly tried to settle. Oh, Shirley, I thought, all mothers feel like this, don't they? They always ask if the baby's all right and check it has the right number of fingers and toes before they even ask if it's a girl or a boy. And so I talked myself to sleep.

The next morning I watched a strip of ceiling move past as I was wheeled into the labour room for an induction. My legs were strapped uncomfortably and inelegantly into high stirrups at the direction of my gynaecologist. Here's a fine thing, I mused. From his angle I must look like Humpty Dumpty, or those female legs suspended in space in a painting by Max Ernst. And from my angle I looked and felt like those stripped, bloodless white meat carcasses hooked by the legs, stiffly hanging in butchers' windows. I hated the sight. I was mildly aware of the unscreened window and wondered if I could be observed, but by now my calves were beginning to ache and I simply wished they would get on with it.

I was alone for a while and beginning to feel rather cold and exposed. I looked about me, at the sickly green paint and, directly above me, at the unnecessary glare of a theatre light. I bet you've seen some sights, I thought, vaguely amused. My gaze rested on the tray of shiny kidney-shaped dishes containing the various instruments ... scalpels, scissors, hooks that always make me grit my teeth and go goose-pimply. My bedside companion was a huge cigar of an oxygen tube, his expressionless dial of a face emotionless, his chipped paint and ugly mask and tubes vaguely reptilian. Gowned figures approached at last. The gynaecologist I could easily recognise but all I could discern of sister was a wisp of grey hair truant from her cap and her inscrutable eyes. Who is she, I thought? Perhaps we're really running a TV serial and we'll all sigh with relief when the director says 'cut' and we'll return to our before-selves and, over coffee, will analyse the scene. This is not a single experience but is derived from my intense training at drama school in London, leading a chameleon life. I was living several lives at any one period ... the young woman from the provinces frightened and alone in London's millions: the sophisticated long-haired student learning quickly to cope with life in the big city; roles from Wesker, Chekhov, Shakespeare and Shaw. It was difficult at times to recognise myself among so many.

In that other theatrical green room with its carnival of colours, masks and grease paint, fantasy and reality emulsified. Even now, when I look at old people I want to yell, 'Right, that's it, that'll do for today' and they'll straighten up, put down their walking sticks, peel off their false noses and wrinkles, wash out the white hair powder, and their youthful step will replace the faltering.

The ageing gynaecologist leaned towards me, the induction hook held like a conductor's baton in his hand, and I thought, Christ, this is for real. 'Now relax, my dear, this may hurt just a little but nothing to worry about,' he soothed. His face, vertical, appeared disproportionate to mine on the horizontal, as in the dentist's chair, when peering at the enlarged pores on his nose, the odd pimple, hairs up his nostrils, and my image in his glasses.

My reflections came to an abrupt end. Ouch! 'Sorry, my dear,' he said as he proceeded, delicately, hook after hook. It was a mildly painful and unnatural experience. Beads of perspiration appeared on his forehead as he worked deftly. We were awaiting a gush of foetal fluid but nothing happened. The doctors exchanged glances. The gynaecologist ceased and the others moved away, discussing earnestly. The ageing one returned to me and said: 'There is no foetal fluid – we may have to perform a caesarean section.'

Get my baby out. Oh God, just get him out, I thought. 'Oh, but you can never be quite sure, you know, my dear,' he went on. 'We'll leave it a few hours and *see* if labour begins spontaneously.' I was returned to my room but I didn't want to be alone and wandered out, discovering the sunroom at the end of the corridor. Another young woman was pacing the floor and I learned that we were, so to speak, in the same boat. 'I'm damned if I'll have a caesarean,' she said. 'I'll move it, you see if I don't. Keep walking, just keep on bloody walking.' So *we* paced the room together and talked hour after hour. It helped, sharing our experience. Towards the evening I began to feel ill and was violently sick. Then the pains began, ruthless and persistent. I had read many books, including Natural Childbirth, helping to prepare myself, and so back in the labour room I panted and counted and panted and counted, trying to control the crescendos of pain. I sucked greedily at the oxygen mask and when my face wasn't crushed to its rubber embrace, I screamed. But the nurse kept pulling it away, leaving me as helpless as a diver struggling in the depths of an ocean. The room was green, the theatre gowns green, the masks and caps green, and I felt trapped in a tank fighting for air, thrashing in pain like a creature harpooned through the navel. The theatre light, a moon reflected through water, wavered and stared relentlessly. I could no longer control the person I had been before I entered this room and, as the hours dragged into the night, I howled like an animal.

One kind Irish nurse stayed with me all night, wiped my brow and crooned to me as only the Irish can. Even now I recall so vividly the intensity of pain and finally, after cuts and a difficult instrument delivery, the ecstasy of release as Anthony was born.

It was just before 6 a.m. Thursday, December 2, 1971. 'It's a boy, my dear,' said the Irish nurse. 'Don't you worry now. He's a beauty to be sure. The two of you just need a good rest now.' Exhausted, I gazed at my baby, all purple and wrinkled as a prune and my tears of relief screened his departure to the nursery. I was even rather amused by the nonchalant chat through my thighs while the gynaecologist sat like some little shoemaker stitching my incisions. 'Right, that's that, my dear,' he said and away I was wheeled into the room already occupied by the two other mums. We soon made friends. Pat had a nine-pound boy and a similar experience to mine and was uncomfortably seated on an air ring. I tried one but found my hip more comfortable.

Now I felt marvellous, despite the soreness, and we could even laugh at our painful attempts to walk to the loo. We were quickly returned to our beds and told not to move. Mary, a pretty Greek girl, had a six-pound girl, delicate as a doll, a textbook delivery and no discomfort at all. Pat and I were really incredulous. We got on famously and at visiting time that evening, with the proud fathers, grandparents, bouquets of flowers and an extra dozen or so wonderfully jovial, chattering Greeks, the room was bursting with love and common joy, until Sister discovered the party and, like a protective mother hen, shooed out the visitors and settled us for the night. Our babies had to be in special for 24 hours so were brought to us for the first time the next morning.

I held my little son in my arms, gazed at his tufts of thick dark hair, at every detail of this new little person, and then placed my little finger in his palm and felt the pressure of his hand on mine. I just couldn't believe it. I really had a son, a nine-pound boy with fists like a boxer. I laughed out loud, thinking of all my foolish fears. I wanted to stand on a rooftop and yell my joy to the world. Then Sister began the first attempt at breast-feeding. As she placed her hands on Anthony's head, guiding his mouth to my breast, he began to cry, his lower jaw trembling violently.

I felt suddenly chilled. There's something wrong with him. There is, there is, I sobbed in desperation as she bundled him into her arms. 'Nonsense, you both need a little more rest,' she said and took Anthony away.

That night he had a brain haemorrhage and I wasn't to see him again until one day several weeks later when I fled from the sight.

As dawn broke the sun's first rays enhanced the pallor of my face, fixed like a mask against the pillows, my hands clutching Anthony's baptism certificate. The vicar had left; he had tried to offer words of comfort but I had barely noticed his entrance and exit. Just the words … 'I have christened your son Anthony, in the operating theatre.'

I thought of Ted and Mum as they had been seated beside my bed, each holding my hand, called in the early hours of Saturday morning. They were dishevelled, shocked and pale. Mother told me afterwards that when awakened with a knock on the door in the night, she thought something had happened to me, not the baby. It had triggered tragic memories of her closest friend who died quite unexpectedly from a blood clot soon after the birth of a son.

I crossed the room silently into the shower cubicle and in the midst of a torrent of water, huddled on the tiled floor, rocked to and fro, and howled out my grief. I can't remember how long I sat there or if someone found me; only that propped once again in bed, the screens drawn across the rest of the room, I awaited the face that would speak the words, 'Your son is dead.' While I struggled with the thought of life without my baby, Anthony was battling death. I was to learn later that he died and was resuscitated in theatre. He'd experienced birth and death in just 48 hours, having crossed the great unknown and returned. I firmly believe that he now knows what that world is beyond and was returned to this one for a purpose.

Chapter 2

The neurosurgeon came shortly after the operation, explaining that he had removed a large blood clot from the surface of Anthony's brain. He was kind, yet frank. He did not think my baby would survive and, if he did, he explained that he would possibly be spastic, blind, deaf and mentally retarded.

'Why did you do it?' I quietly asked. I asked you to leave him alone.

I did not want any visitors. I could not eat, and the slightest noise was an unbearable irritant. I left the hospital and returned to the flat we were renting while our home was being built, the home for our son. I stayed in the bedroom, the drapes drawn to shut out the light, as if night had been drawn across my world. I did not wish to see Anthony. I wanted to remember him as he was, so beautiful the few moments I had held him in my arms.

One morning the strident ring of the telephone split the silence. I was alone and resented the intrusion. It was the ward sister asking me when I was coming to see Anthony. I made some excuse and slammed down the receiver, but each day she phoned until, reluctantly, I agreed to go. I trembled as the lift droned upwards to the top floor to Rose Ward. I wanted it to go on and on and never stop, to remain in that impersonal box forever.

Even before I pushed through the doors into the ward, I could see him, my baby, my beautiful boy, now a grey emaciated scrap in his incubator, barely breathing. I stared at the naked little body, his left side now rigidly spastic and his bald plastered head bereft of its once luxuriant dark hair. I bent and kissed him through the glass case, then fled from the room, down and round, down and round, flight after flight of stairs, spiralling in panic, to escape from the horror of his suffering. Miraculously, Anthony clung to life and began to gain weight. When he was removed from the incubator into a cot the sister called me again. 'He's a dear little man,' were her last words as I put the receiver down. The words hung in the air. … 'He's a dear little man.' I looked at the beautiful photograph taken of Anthony, aged 24 hours, before his ordeal began. I hadn't even known that all the babies were photographed. Mine had been sent on by the photographer. There was his thick dark hair, his crinkly face, eyes closed, and those two lovely large hands clenched to fists, almost as if he knew a battle was ahead of him. If he survived, I thought, if by some quirk of fate he is not going to be all those ghastly things predicted by the neurosurgeon, he could just grow up to be a man. I grabbed my handbag and dashed to the hospital.

The paediatrician said the signs were encouraging. Anthony was feeding normally and had a good cry. I thought, a cry is a cry. But later experience in these baby wards was to reveal that the seriously brain-damaged child has a chilling, heart rending high-pitched wailing. My dear little man was doing so well. Each day I went eagerly to the hospital to learn to bath and feed him. I know it sounds strange saying 'learn,' but to touch him when he looked so frail and to actually bathe his little head rimmed with scars needed the encouragement, kindness and expertise of the duty sisters. Rose Ward had several new born babies such as Anthony, and I watched their struggles to survive, too.

On Christmas Day, while feeding Anthony, two babies arrived in humidicribs and were placed on either side of Anthony's cot. One, a cherub of a boy, had stopped breathing in the ambulance and was now apparently severely brain damaged. He was also a child who would have been up for adoption. I cried openly. I was beginning to be awed by the life within these walls. And the death.

This little boy was born and died and was reborn on Christmas Day, and now no-one would adopt him because of his brain damage. This tiny, lovely baby would grow into an institutionalised automaton. I wondered which was the greater tragedy, this or the other baby boy whose face had no features. But he did have loving, caring parents. Across the room I noticed a pretty baby girl with unusually long black hair and huge dark eyes. Her name was Rita and she and Anthony were to spend some considerable time together.

About a month after his birth, when I came to see Anthony one morning, I noticed a lump on his back. Checking his chart, I saw he had vomited his early morning feed and had a little diarrhoea. When the paediatrician came on his rounds immediate action followed and once again Anthony was prepared for surgery. He had haemorrhaged in the region of the left kidney, possibly at the same time as his initial brain haemorrhage. This smaller and undetected one had developed into an abscess. Critically ill, Anthony again was given little hope of survival. This second blow was harder to bear. For days now I had gradually grown to love and accept and care for my son. The first time I was told he wouldn't live I didn't know him. I had even rejected him to protect myself from the pain of losing him, as if I had erected a thick glass barrier between us.

Those first days in his incubator I had been able to see him but not touch him or hold him close. He was a part of me yet a stranger to me. Now he was my son he had an identity, and the thought of losing him was unbearable.

This time, while he was in theatre, I was sitting beside his cot waiting and praying for his return, desperately willing him to live again. My valiant little man pulled through, but he was too ill even to nurse. A sister ushered me away home, saying I would be of no use to him exhausted and distraught.

As Ted slept, I stared into the darkness. My baby's going to die and I've just got to come to terms with it, I thought. I've always said I've wanted a normal healthy son, and not a spastic, possibly a mentally retarded one, haven't I? Always been adamant that the quality of life is paramount, that I couldn't cope with a brain-damaged child or see the point. On and on, question and answer in my head, I was trying to cushion myself for the finality of Anthony's death.

Later, being alone in the flat was a nightmare of recriminations. I spent my time going over and over my pregnancy. Had I done something that had harmed Anthony? Was I in some way guilty of causing this tragedy?

I went to the hospital and stayed all day, but Anthony didn't know me. He was having frequent convulsions and would stop breathing and be so very still, it seemed I was witnessing his death over and over again. I felt raw with misery. It was apparent that Anthony would be hospitalised some considerable time if he survived, so I decided to return to teaching.

I had spent many years teaching both in England and Australia. I began teaching in Harlow New Town in Essex, not an easy area to start a new profession. I had to deal with many problem children, uprooted mainly from the poorer areas of London and set down like aliens on another planet in this new town of concrete, brick and plastic. It was hard work. But once accepted by the children, seeing their interest grow was reward enough. I found there was a great need for youth workers and I became involved several nights each week taking drama groups at the youth centre. We also organised residential courses at youth centres established in Essex. These were mainly large old Georgian or Victorian houses given to the organisation for youth, and we were able to involve these youngsters in many courses. Later, I purposely chose to teach in the East End of London in a large comprehensive school. We had a divided catchment area, one section relatively affluent, the other a huge impersonal housing estate. I taught literature to the higher streamed classes, which was immensely satisfying. I was also responsible for the school drama festival and productions and in this way came in contact with many more children than my allotted classes. We rehearsed each evening after school. I enjoyed the company of my colleagues and arranged trips to Italy, France and Spain, accompanying children fortunate enough to have parents who could afford holidays for them. Most of all I enjoyed the challenge of the so-called difficult classes, especially the school-leavers, tough 15-year-old boys and girls reared in a tough environment. The statistics were high of children from problem families, broken homes, foster homes and those on probation. Each of those youngsters became special to me and I remember them with affection. It was as if I had a huge family, and I spent my days and most evenings and many school holidays with children. I can see that being with so many vibrant youngsters I never really felt the need to have children of my own. It was only after several years of teaching that I decided I would like to broaden my horizons and leave teaching for a while.

Chapter 3

I decided to drive overland to Australia, the famous London to Sydney route. I had many Australian colleagues I had met in England.

It was during my preparation for the first stage of this journey that I met Ted. We were both floundering from broken marriages. Ted was living with his sister, and I with an old college friend, Freida and her two children. I had filed for divorce several months previously, then given up my job teaching and decided I was going to drive through Europe. I especially wanted to stay in Rome to study the architecture, then drive down to Brindisi, ship across to Patris in Greece and join friends touring in the Greek theatre company to learn more about classical Greek drama.

My meeting with Ted was only eight days before my departure. I was travelling alone. I wanted to be alone … 'to pick up the pieces' is the expression most commonly used. My husband was away on a business trip and I returned to our home to collect the rest of my belongings. I decided to spend that evening saying goodbye at our club. Ted regularly sang there but I had never before spoken with him. This particular evening he joined a group of my friends and we were introduced.

It was one of those rare occasions when two people meet and instantly feel they have a great deal in common. We chatted about my proposed trip and Ted was keenly interested to learn that from Athens I eventually planned to go to Australia to reunite with Australian colleagues who had been teaching for a year at my school in London. Two days past and he telephoned and invited me out for a drink. He said he had always wanted to go to Australia but had never been able to persuade his wife to leave her mother. I said if he was interested he could join me in Athens as I would welcome a co-driver on the overland trip to Australia. It didn't trouble me to drive to Athens alone, but I knew it would be foolish to contemplate travelling further east. He said he would prefer I delay my departure so that we could leave together. I asked him if he was sure he wanted to make such a journey and if he was absolutely certain that he could not be reconciled with his family. Apparently the marriage had been precarious for some time.

I traded my car for a Land Rover and hectic days were spent tramping from one embassy to another for visas. Cholera and typhoid shots were needed so we chose alternate arms, fortunately. The first ones were extremely painful and caused fever, delirium and swollen useless arms. I remember we drove through London bound for Europe, Ted steering with his good arm and me changing gear with mine.

We travelled through Greece to Turkey, across the Bosphorus to Istanbul and on into Iran. We were attacked several times by bandits. Ted and I became very close struggling through such adventures, battling rugged mountains and spending endless days on sizzling desert roads, marvelling at the snow-capped Himalayas on our left and the folds of velvet hills ahead. We saw camel trains, the black tents of nomads, strange stilt houses by the Black Sea and the domed mud-dwellings in the interior, the veiled ghostlike inhabitants disappearing as we approached.

In our struggle and adventure we had to live, work and sleep together. The Land Rover was our security and home and we fell in love, enjoying this adventure together. Week after week we were in a world of our own and while we were crossing the deserts we didn't even know that man had walked on the moon.

Gradually our food ran out and in Eastern Iran for three weeks we lived only on chapatti, raw onion, and watermelon. In Kandahar, Afghanistan, thin and ravenous, we teamed up with a Kombi-van of young Americans inevitably heading for Katmandu. We filled a small cafe and ate whatever it was unquestioningly. A boy was employed to keep the black ceiling flies on the move and kick away the rats at the same time.

We tailed unbelievably ancient convoys of brightly painted trucks through the jagged and austere Khyber Pass, a colossal graveyard of memorial stones to British soldiers who fought and died there.

We travelled on to Delhi in India, where we sold our gear to an Australian architect and ended our overland trip because of riots in India and guerrilla attacks in Burma.

We flew out of Delhi with barely more than our tickets to Darwin and arrived in Australia's northern capital at night in November, the wet season. Stepping out of the plane was like stepping into a sauna. I felt as if I couldn't breathe. Two days later Ted found a job driving a truck out in the bush and by the next day I was back in school teaching. After paying two weeks rent in advance on a bed sitter, we were left with only $8. We didn't eat for the first week but laughed because we had actually made it to Australia and Ted said: 'Well, we are at rock bottom now, we can only climb upwards.' I remember the pleasure of our first cold beer on Ted's payday in a bar in Smith Street and our disbelieving laughter as a purple-black Aborigine danced on a table-top without her knickers on.

It was all strange, new and exciting. A fresh life had begun for us in Australia. We had each other and sharing such a journey we had become very, very close. We made many good friends, worked and saved hard and loved Darwin for the two years we were there.

Then I conceived and it seemed our happiness was complete. We made plans to move south to Adelaide and arrived there in November, 1971. We took a flat and planned our home together for our child, and a new future. Our plans shattered around the tragedy of Anthony.

Chapter 4

I had for so long been such a close part of Anthony's world that I now felt the compulsion to return to the world of normal, healthy children and to try, at least for part of each day, to forget all those tragic, suffering little ones at the hospital who had for some inexplicable reason been so cruelly cheated of life's potential. I taught literature at high school, mainly school certificate and matriculation English. I approached my work with a superhuman enthusiasm. Up early each morning, I marked books or prepared lessons, choosing special poems or literary excerpts from my own books for duplication where books were not available in school. Eagerly I looked forward to arriving at school, entering into the atmosphere of the staffroom exchange of repartee, the camaraderie and the chat over coffee before the full day ahead when the school bell rang.

I knew I would be too busy to dwell on the fact that none of my children were really mine at all. How differently I now viewed the rows of heads before me. I had always respected individuality, but I now saw each child as part of two other human beings, and I understood with greater clarity just how many different emotions can come from such a combination … the love, hate, cruelty, jealousy, heartache, ambition and pride of both parents and children. I was aware that the demands on my time, energy and intellect kept me from dwelling on the most useless and destructive of emotions – self-pity.

The contrast of each day was devastating. I moved from the bustle of healthy, active children at school to the world of the sick ones at the hospital and each became special to me but in a different way. I gave my all to my students and they in turn gave to me their affection, interest and vitality, which helped balance the other world of the inactive, debilitated ones. Each became an adopted family to fill the aching void of my childless home.

As I neared the hospital I felt Anthony's presence. I dreaded seeing him in agony but longed to be with him. When I had spent all day every day with him, I found it too much. Now I felt as if I had been charged with vitality during my working day, which I could now share with him.

He was not alone. Mother had come over from England for Anthony's birth and a holiday which had turned into a nightmare. She never left us. Her quiet love and support had carried me through the initial horror of Anthony's first few weeks of life, and now she spent every day at the hospital by his side, talking to him and nursing him when possible, when he was not attached to transfusions, and sitting with him for hours pouring out tremendous love for her grandchild.

As a toddler, and even now, years later, Anthony prefers Nanna's songs, those World War Two songs so appropriate during his struggle to live. I took over at four o'clock and stayed until his 10 o'clock feed, then it was home to bed and up early to prepare for school. I knew that somehow, I must keep busy to anaesthetise the past months. It was during that in-between time, before sleep blotted out the day, I allowed myself to think ... to contemplate the reality of the future and what it would hold. That time was sheer hell. Anthony had now been moved from the surgical ward into Princess Ward, and in the adjacent cot was Rita. No diagnosis had been given for Anthony's condition, and I knew only what I had been told by the neurosurgeon and paediatrician that Anthony had an abnormally low platelet count. Platelets are the clotting agents in the blood, so that his immediate threat of death was by haemorrhaging. I also knew that Anthony was critically anaemic, but I thought this was due to his massive haemorrhages. It meant frequent blood transfusions to keep him alive. When he was not fixed to a blood transfusion Mother and I worked continuously on his spastic side, placing his dummy and a soft toy or rattle in his feet so that he had to lift his legs and use his hands to reach for what he wanted. Soon he was able to use his limbs almost normally.

Apart from the unsightly eczema and the shaven head, we were pleased with his physical improvement. At one period after his second haemorrhage and operation I feared he had defective sight, as he would avert his eyes from any bright light, and I noticed one pupil dilated more than the other. We had to screen his cot even from the daylight. But later I knew he could see when he reacted with a smile when we appeared.

We were not alone in our evening vigils. Rita was initially admitted with thrush, a fungus infection which had later spread to her lungs. The struggle to feed her and to keep her respiratory tract open was weakening her. Her parents, a southern European couple, arrived shortly after I did. The father, obviously having come straight from work, rushed to wash his hands and don his gown to nurse his baby daughter. He would sing to Rita, very softly. I didn't understand the words, but language was no barrier to their meaning. Our faces mirrored our thoughts well enough.

One Saturday morning as I entered the ward and reached for my gown I noticed Rita's cot was empty. She was in theatre for heart surgery. Her mother sat quietly by her cot, waiting, as I had once waited for Anthony. But Rita never returned. I just couldn't believe it. This was my first experience of knowing a child who died. I have since witnessed many more such tragic deaths ... they don't become any easier to bear. Each is still brought sharply into focus. I can see Rita even now as she was those evenings, alive in her cot a few feet away from Anthony.

Driving home, and later when I went to bed early, leaving Ted and Mum watching TV, I reflected upon Rita's death and Anthony's death. My initial rejection of him filled me with horror. All right, you say you knew what would happen, you had a premonition, even visualised the scene in your mind's eye. But how could you surrender your son with such emphatic immediacy? My other me would answer, but you have seen schools for handicapped children, you have even taught low-IQ children. As a student you favoured euthanasia, thought it wrong to prolong potentially useless lives; such a colossal financial drain, when there are so many normal, would-be healthy children born into the Third World who simply die from a lack of food and water. I lived near an asylum as a child and could, in the distance, see those pathetic figures shuffling around in the grounds in their twilight world. I didn't want this for my son. To grow old without me.

I thought of my horror as a child at the sight of a little boy with a grotesque head dragging back his thin white neck like a huge apple on a rope; it was hydrocephalus, now relatively easily treated. I remember the school bus crowded with mongoloid children that waited beside ours and the cruelty of some of my peers, mocking them by pulling and slanting their eyes and sticking their tongues against the windows. I averted my face; puzzling even then the why of it all.

Now, after my experience with these different ones and their struggle at life's beginning, I do not feel revulsion and certainly not pity. I silently applaud their immense courage at accepting life's challenge, invariably with more zest and success than some of their so-called normal contemporaries. I thought that without experience no one could coldly discuss statistics, done with such equanimity by our bureaucrats. But we are not statistics. We are all individuals. With realisation I spoke aloud: 'Anthony is an individual and has all the rights of an individual; he has survived so far. Perhaps he has the guts to make it.'

For the first time for many a long night I fell asleep quickly, planning the future for our son. But Anthony began rapidly deteriorating. Test followed test. He had haemorrhaged from the bowels, the bladder, the nose and into his skin, leaving his body covered with delicate mottled purple marks and ugly black bruises. One transfusion followed another. Each limb was marked with tiny scars left from the incisions, until the only place left to transfuse him was his head. I entered that winter's evening to witness the full impact of my baby's suffering. It was then I cried: ENOUGH.

I felt it was both selfish and cruel to keep Anthony alive, to prolong his life of such suffering. I would willingly have died for my little son. How many nights had I cried silently, 'Dear God, spare him and take me.'

As Anthony was approaching the age of six months his complex condition was finally diagnosed: Wiskott-Aldrich Syndrome, a rare bone marrow disease. 'His condition is incurable,' stated the paediatrician. 'I'm afraid children rarely survive beyond the age of two years.' We were sitting in a small consulting room next to the ward, and the paediatrician was kind and concerned. I had come to know and respect him. Perhaps he thought I was going to scream in protest, at least burst into tears ... something. But the single word INCURABLE had ruthless finality and suspended me in disbelief.

To me the word INCURABLE meant a living death, a horrific waiting for the inevitable. We all know we must die eventually, but it's something we tend to push to the back of our minds, something we expect to happen at the end of our days, not at the beginning. The death of an ageing relative is a heart rending loss, but the death of a child is a tragedy which seems so pointless. To crave and give life and to end it so abruptly ... it's like shutting out the sun. I wondered how I would continue to live knowing my only child was dying. In the night I alternately prayed and bartered for Anthony's life.

I suffered really bad times, torn with inadequacy and helplessness, when I cursed the Lord and tears scoured my eyes to blood-red sockets.

The next evening Ted, mother and I were with Anthony, mother nursing him. We were gowned and masked to protect him from infection. 'He's very hot,' said mother. Just feel his head; I'm sure he has a temperature.' I called the nurse who discovered Anthony's temperature had soared to 103. The paediatrician took Ted and me to one side. 'I believe now is the time to let nature take its course, and not administer antibiotics,' he said.

He was, in fact, advising euthanasia, the withdrawing of supporting drugs or transfusions. He left us alone to decide. I was bitter and speechless. A lump in my throat as large as an apple was stemming a well of tears. Let nature take its course …? Hadn't I asserted this all along? They had operated, resuscitated Anthony; pumped pint after pint of blood into him; covered him with scars; caused him indescribable pain; and now, let nature takes its course!

Six months ago, before I had come to know my little son as a person in his own right, how much easier that decision could have been made. We had already tried to prepare ourselves for this time. We held hands, our eyes met. Words were unnecessary. We had made our decision. Our little son had suffered enough.

Chapter 5

The paediatrician said Anthony was now in no pain but would survive only about three weeks without blood transfusions. He assured us that being so anaemic he would sleep more and more and would die very peacefully. We drove home in silence, each lost in our own thoughts. I kept saying to myself that it was the kindest thing to do … the only decision to make. But another part of me was screaming, NO! We gathered round the fire and began quietly talking. Soon we were openly weeping, Ted, mother and I. Anthony had incredibly survived for six months only to be diagnosed incurable.

I was the last to go to bed. I turned out the lights, standing alone in the hallway. I simply stood there in the blackness. Then, by some indefinable compulsion, I dropped to my knees and placed my forehead on the floor and with arms stretched out, palms crossed, I prayed … not for a peaceful death for my baby, but as I have never done before, for my baby to live. My forehead radiated heat, the blackness of my head turned to a fiery red, and the pressure of my closed lids became sparks of vivid yellow. The next morning I viewed with incredulity my experience of the night before. Basically agnostic, I had earnestly appealed to God for my son's life.

With resignation I gathered together some of Anthony's beautiful unused clothes in preparation for our final journey to the hospital to bring him home to die. The paediatrician had tried to dissuade us from this decision; he feared that we would not be able to cope. But as I stood looking at the empty cot, the nursery planned with such love, the untouched teddy bear propped against the tiny pillow, and at the little jacket in my hand, I knew I wanted our baby home.

He had known only pain and constant hospitalisation, the touch of many kind hands, but the hands of strangers. I wanted to pour a lifetime of love into the short time he would be with us in his home, with his family about him; to cradle him in my arms, singing to him as he drifted into eternal sleep. I had now come to believe in the right to die with dignity for young and old alike. I did not then consider with such fervour the right to live, as I do now. On the way to the hospital to collect Anthony, poor mother was racked with sobs, but I was quiet and thoughtful. 'No more tears, Mum,' I said quietly. 'We must not surround Anthony with sorrow but love and joy in his last days.'

Once again the paediatrician called Ted and me into the consulting room while mother nursed Anthony. 'His temperature is down,' he said, 'and he's had a peaceful night and I've spent a disturbed evening considering every aspect of his case. I am going to try him with steroid drugs.'

'Will it cause him any more pain?' was all I could ask. I was stunned at this reversal of all we had been prepared for. 'No, it is a cortisone drug and could help his condition,' the specialist replied.

Anthony remained in hospital, incredibly requiring no further blood transfusions. I was later to realise the power of this drug, the benefits, and the ghastly side effects.

* * *

At eight months we were able to take Anthony home, supported by this drug. He looked so plump, bonny and healthy it was difficult to accept the reality of his condition. Each day I would push the inevitable to the back of my mind. I marked 12 months on the pantry wall, crossing off the eight past, and on the second of each ensuing month I crossed one out, marking another month Anthony had survived.

I continued teaching, just to the end of the school term, as mother had to return to England. Her original holiday trip to Australia for Anthony's birth had stretched into almost a year. She had shared the constant love and care of her grandson. Sobbing quietly, she bent and kissed the sleeping Anthony goodbye as she left for home. Caring for Anthony was an exacting task without mother's support. He would awake, programmed each hour throughout the night, corresponding with his hourly temperatures in hospital. I became tired and irritable through lack of sleep. The house had to be kept meticulously clean. Anthony's eczema was aggravated by dust. Never having particularly liked housework, what would be an average weekly cleaning up in a normal house with normal children was a daily chore and a drain on my time and energy. Everything Anthony used I sterilised in Milton solution, and if that wasn't possible wiped disinfectant over his playthings and surfaces with which he came in contact to protect him from infection. We discouraged visitors entering the house, always a potential infection risk, and began the procedure of removing our outdoor shoes in the laundry and changing into clean ones. We were simulating his barrier nursing as much as possible. But the days had their moments of joy. When I took him for walks round the perimeter of the creek where we lived he enjoyed the splendour of the lofty bluegums, the flocks of galahs decorating their boughs like huge pink blossoms; the sunlight through the leaves, and the laugh of the kookaburra.

Each sunny day I would place him on the front lawn on a blanket with his toys, and neighbours' children would come and talk to him. He was not in physical contact. It was enough for him to raise his face to the sun and laugh with them. I continued to massage his limbs and spent hour after hour each day playing games, making him laugh, clapping hands and feet together, alternately up and down, side to side to strengthen the muscles until the day when he could hold a ball in both hands, even hold his bottle and drink by himself; then, examine and experiment with both hands any tiny new toy. I waited for the day of triumph when he would stand unaided and fight to make those first steps. He was not blind, he was not deaf. He could sit, walk and respond brightly, and I think our greatest reward was his first words of Mumma, Nanna and Daddy.

Although Anthony would allow me to gently touch and massage his body he never would allow me to stroke his head, and sadly I couldn't even kiss him because I feared passing on germs. I would frequently gargle with Listerine, hoping to be as antiseptic as possible. There was always this invisible barrier between us. I took Anthony for regular check-ups to the Adelaide Children's Hospital, but he was doing so well he was taken off the steroid drugs. Anthony's first birthday at home was a day of shared love and warmth. Being one year old is rather special, but for Anthony it was a milestone, a day of triumph for him and for all of us. We had a birthday cake with a single flickering candle enhancing the glow of joy on our faces as we watched Anthony play with his birthday toys. Two especially he adored ... Woof, a bizarre lime-green dog and Pinky, a musical pig on a round base, his daytime favourites and his night-time companions. He always held them close as he fell asleep. They have accompanied him to and fro from hospital so many times, and he still has those now rather bedraggled and patched friends six plus years later.

* * *

For a while everything seemed so normal that I began to relax more and for the first time enjoy my home and my baby until one crisp autumn morning. I was washing the breakfast dishes. Anthony was playing on the lounge carpet when I heard a choking sound. I ran the few feet to him.

He looked as if he had been brutally beaten. His face and front were bright red and spreading out round him like a matador's cloak lay a pool of blood. It was as if his tiny body was emptying, spilling out blood from his nose and mouth so rapidly that he was gasping to breathe.

From the time I had accepted Anthony in those early weeks I had remained so calm, always trying to mask my feelings. I never cried in front of Anthony. I always sobbed in private, usually in the shower.

Yet this time I was panic stricken. I ran outside and yelled for Erica, my neighbour on one side and screamed for Jenny on the other. It was Jenny who ran in and quickly called Peter, our next-door-but-one neighbour. I bundled Anthony into a towel, grabbing an extra one to stem the blood flow and my tears, and while Peter and I sped to the Children's Hospital, Jenny not only coped with cleaning the massive bloodstain, but with Peter's wife who had fainted.

Anthony had an infection which had depleted his already abnormally low clotting cells, causing a haemorrhage. He bled for seven hours and then ceased. Exhausted, snuffling with his blood-clotted nostrils, the poor little chap slept, back once again in his isolation cubicle. This was to happen more and more as he approached the age of one and a half years. So many days the neighbours rallied to help, so many nights Ted and I, who now took it in turns to sleep in Anthony's room, would call each other for the race through the night to the hospital.

Anthony's deterioration was rapid and horrific. He bled profusely from the nose, swallowing large amounts of blood which made him vomit bright red. He bled into his skin causing the purple mottling, and his little body was a patchwork of ugly dark bruises.

Even worse were the haemorrhages from the bowels and bladder until the laundry was filled with bloodstained nappies soaking in buckets, pink like wine.

We would hear him snuffling in the night and find him lying soaked in blood in his cot. This invariably happened more during the night and the journey to hospital, the examination, the bright lights, the isolation cubicle again and again only increased his distress and lengthened the haemorrhage time. I began to accept and to cope with his haemorrhages. I had to, for Anthony's sake.

These frequent rushes to. the hospital, I realised, achieved little except to release me for a while from the horror and fatigue of dealing with the haemorrhage. The staff were wonderfully efficient and kind but there was nothing really that could be done for Anthony in hospital. I would lift him from his cot and bathe his face with a cool cloth and then, semi-upright, nurse him and sing to him, first to calm him, and then to keep him gently and frequently swabbed so he could breathe more easily. I would note the length of bleeding and assess the blood loss. I knew now by experience just how long to keep him at home. Hour after hour in the night I paced the floor, soothing my blooded infant until I felt my limbs would snap with fatigue. But it was all worthwhile as invariably it did decrease the blood loss and Anthony's distress.

As the effects of the steroid drugs wore off Anthony's eczema returned. I could not use soap on him and had to bathe him in Condy's crystals which stained him brown, creating a bizarre and unsightly combination of bruised, mottled and scratched flesh. His scalp peeled and I had to coat it with cream so that his hair stood up in peaks like miniature Christmas trees, an unbearable irritant for him in the warm weather. It was heartbreaking watching him become weaker and weaker, critically anaemic.

We were preparing ourselves again for his last days; he was pale blue and listless and slept for long periods. So many times I stood by his cot to check that he was still breathing, until the crescendo of sounds from my own pulse thundered in my ears and made the detection of his fluttering heartbeat impossible.

I just couldn't relate this changed little boy to the little lad cheering on his swing out on the patio or splashing in his wading pool in the sunshine just a few weeks previously.

On the eve of Good Friday, 1973, after a day of watching Anthony's struggle to live, I vividly recall lying in my darkened room and silently, desperately calling to the Lord once more to spare my son. Lord, he's an innocent, he has suffered so much and yet is without sin; punish me, I am the sinner. He has struggled so valiantly to live. He died and you returned him to me. I don't understand. The sins of the father are visited on the son ... those words flashed as bright as any neon sign in my mind. But that isn't just. A God of love? Where is this God of love? I cried. How can He watch little children suffer and die?

I became aware of a presence in the room, a powerful aura, but I was not afraid. I felt only a great calm in answer.

* * *

The following morning as we were seated for breakfast, Jenny, my next-door neighbour, came in with a few lines clipped out of the Adelaide Advertiser, about a bone marrow transplant on a little boy of Anthony's age in London. It was at the Westminster Hospital and the boy was Simon Bostic. It briefly mentioned his condition which sounded remarkably similar to Anthony's. I wrote immediately to Mrs Bostic and phoned the Westminster Hospital where I spoke directly to Professor Humble, who had carried out the implant, and explained my son's condition. I remember those words echoing from 12,000 miles into my receiver: 'We've done it once, we can do it again.' A coincidence, fate, or response to prayer?

With this breakthrough in medical science in 1973, my son, born in 1971 incurable, was now possibly curable. Events occurred, with contacts from the press, with the force of a blast from an exploding zeppelin. Sydney, Melbourne and Adelaide called and reporters were on my doorstep. The first Press photograph of Anthony appeared on the front page of the Adelaide Advertiser. He was at our large lounge window staring out at a winter's morning.

The first step was to have all our family in Australia tissue-typed for compatibility with Anthony's cells in order to donate some of our bone marrow for his transplant. The doctors in Adelaide expressed caution, as the little boy in England had granulomatous, not Wiskott-Aldrich Syndrome.

Caution be damned, I thought, gritting my teeth, we've nothing to lose. My son is supposedly incurable, and this is the first glimmer of hope, and while ever there is a chance that Anthony can live I'll go to the corners of the earth, let alone London.

My mind was in a turmoil. The doctors told me I was clutching at straws. London seemed disinclined to give positive directives and

I couldn't even learn the results of our blood tests. I desperately sought help. I approached the South Australian State Premier Don Dunstan for assistance; neighbours petitioned our local MP Molly Byrne. I even contacted and received replies from the Federal Minister of Health and Prime Minister Gough Whitlam, but little help was available for Anthony and others like him in Australia. The story had spread Australia-wide as well as internationally and, bless them, some miners in Coober Pedy, an opal-mining town in the outback of South Australia, offered to pay our fares to England. Time was passing rapidly so I demanded the results of our blood tests. Mother's was identical with Anthony's. She had returned to Australia, once she knew of the renewed hope for Anthony, to assist me to fly with him to London. Simultaneously, a directive had been issued from the doctors in London saying that they would accept Anthony only on condition of a total publicity ban. It meant we were unable to accept the offer from Coober Pedy. To begin with I was terrified if the phone rang or a knock came at the door. I was afraid to speak in case I endangered Anthony's chances. The Press was wonderful. I explained the situation and they remained silent, but, in the interim, Anthony was becoming weaker. Still no positive date to take him to London was proposed. My terror turned to desperate determination. I phoned the editor of the Adelaide Advertiser and discussed our plight. From his office we called London and the editor monitored the call. I felt that the transplant team in London was procrastinating. I was later to realise why. Neither the editor nor I enjoyed what we had to do, but I stressed to the professor on the phone that Anthony was barely alive. I read out Anthony's and mother's identical tissue types. The editor and I had agreed that if Anthony was not flown to London immediately we would break the publicity ban. Incredibly, four months had passed since the day my neighbour brought in the Press clipping. The words 'Fly him in on the next available flight,' was our reply from London.

I scraped every cent together for two air fares, mine and mother's. Ted was to remain in Australia to keep his job to support us while we were away the anticipated six months. Anthony was readmitted to the Adelaide Children's Hospital for another blood transfusion. He was so weak that this was essential if he was to survive such a journey. I was also informed that the high altitude could precipitate more severe haemorrhages. It took 48 hours to make the frenzied arrangements, listen to advice, inform and meet the airline officials and choose the most suitable seating to make the journey as comfortable as possible and to try to ensure Anthony's survival.

The publicity ban held, but I agreed to our departure being photographed, although the photographs were not to be used until our joint agreement. They appeared in the Australian papers months later. I was to find that my often-unknown new friends in the press were my strongest allies in the fight for my son's life.

Chapter 6

That cold August morning in 1973, at Adelaide Airport, the cameras recorded the event as Anthony boarded the plane on our mission of hope. Even before we touched down at Melbourne he had begun to haemorrhage and in the VIP Lounge, with kind help from Qantas, we changed numerous blood-soaked nappies.

I wanted to turn back to Ted, to my home, to all that was familiar and comforting, but the roar of the Jumbo jet engines summoned and I knew I must call on the same sort of power, generated by love, to transport my baby across the world for his chance to live. As the plane soared away its silver wings dipped and reflected the morning light and the shapes of Melbourne receded and blended into the pastel Australia beneath. I saw this physical uplifting as a symbol of hope, my uplifting to carry my own precious cargo with faith and courage, on to Sydney and Bangkok, on and on.

Anthony haemorrhaged and cried, terrified by the noise and the hustle and bustle of the hundreds of travellers on happier journeys than our own. The only time he laughed was at take-off and landing when the thrust of the engines and the tremendous pull-back forced our bodies against our seats.

I had been unable to eat since leaving home because Anthony would not leave my arms. I nursed and nursed him, when possible balancing against the motion of the plane. My mainstay was black coffee. I knew I had to keep awake and alert. Approaching Bahrein he eventually fell asleep. I ached with tension and fatigue. I hadn't dared move for many hours. My thigh, pressed against the outside arm rest, was numb and bruised black. The night was scarred with brilliant forked lightning and the plane plummeted and rose, buffeted in a storm. This violent motion seemed to soothe Anthony to sleep as if he were rocked in a huge cradle in the sky. While other passengers were being sick Anthony, at last, lay peacefully asleep along the seats, held safely by mother kneeling on the floor and protecting him. One of the many kind stewards came and took my place, bringing mother a large brandy while another literally steered me to Captain Cook's Cabin and insisted I partake of the same.

The fiery warmth spread to my stiffened limbs and tense aching neck muscles as I gradually relaxed and stretched with relief. I accepted a cigarette from a lone gentleman, unable to sleep, and discovered we knew friends in Adelaide. With a little more brandy and bonhomie, suspended in time, we shared the storm in the night. As our jet breached the dawn I returned to my seat. The haemorrhages continued and I thought we would never reach London. It was incredible how much blood can come from one little being. The plane was still taxiing at London's Heathrow Airport as I clutched my baby, barely alive, and unsteadily headed for the nearest exit. A nurse speedily climbed the steps and reached for Anthony but I held him close and slowly, carefully, carried him down to the ambulance waiting on the runway. We sped away leaving mother near to exhaustion, but stalwart as ever, to cope with our luggage in the terminal.

I remember arriving at the tiny Westminster Children's Hospital in a narrow side street. Again, the whirr of a lift, again arms to take Anthony, but I held him even more tightly. I felt I was going to faint and asked the ambulance man to hold on to me. Only when Anthony was secure in his cot in the tiny isolation cubicle, 12,000 miles from home, did my arms drop wearily to my sides and I remember no more.

* * *

I awoke in the mothers' unit, dazed and disorientated. I gazed around my room at the cream walls, the single bed, chair and table, and from the faded curtains to the square window and the London sky. 'We've made it,' I sighed. The relief was overwhelming as I drifted off, still rocked by the motion of the plane. When I awoke I desperately wanted reassurance that Anthony was still alive. I fumbled for clothes and staggered out to find him. Anthony was there. He looked so pale, his tiny sleeping form pressed between the sheets. Yet he was alive and I thanked God, humbly.

The tests began on mother and Anthony for compatibility for the bone marrow transplant. Six days we waited for the results. With incredulity and abject disappointment, I listened while the doctors said they had rejected. They even repeated the test simulation and it rejected a second time. Our journey across the world was apparently in vain, but I was determined not to turn back. This was where Anthony could be cured and this was where he would stay, but now another donor must be found if Anthony was to have a chance to live. I was told that the testing of potential donors was continuing. I was not aware that it was only a handful each week.

With Anthony's chances of finding a non-relative donor at 50,000 to one it would, I later calculated, have taken decades to find his 'Mister Right' and by then it would be too late. Yet one day came the tremendous news that a man near Los Angeles, in the United States, had the same tissue type as Anthony. He took some tracking down, as he had moved interstate; finally he was located and Anthony's blood was flown to the United States for compatibility tests. Again the knife-edge pressure, endless days of awaiting results, the intense hoping that this unknown American could save Anthony; and then the shattering disappointment as the results proved incompatible.

The cells of the donor and the recipient must match perfectly or they attack each other. The host can reject the donor cells or the reverse. When the donor attacks the patient's cells it can prove fatal and there are many complex reactions each way which can prove disastrous.

It is a highly complex form of medical treatment, still in the pioneer stages, but it is the result of decades of dedicated research by brilliant doctors and professors. Knowing all this I still wanted to risk this only chance for my son.

Mother had taken a job in the Gordon Hospital, in the next street, to be near Anthony. With the job went a room only a hundred yards from Anthony and me in the Children's Hospital. She even chose to work shifts so that one of us could always be with Anthony.

Our days from early morning to late evening were spent in the cubicle with Anthony to give him love and comfort and to try to make those endless days less empty. When he had gathered a little strength his great grandmother, great aunt, aunties and his uncle came to visit him. It was a long journey from the north of England, and they were only allowed to see him through the windows of the cubicle. He sensed they were not medical staff, that they loved him and he toddled to the door and kissed them one by one through its glass pane.

* * *

It is difficult to describe Anthony's seven months in isolation. It is only now I realise the immense psychological damage to a child deprived of all that is normal, his home, his family and the contact of little ones his own age. He was locked away from the world in a room of glass to protect him from infection, a world with which he could not cope, as if he had been born an alien. He had haemorrhaged so severely he had bled his bowel lining and now would take only fluids, water or blackcurrant juice.

I tried everything to tempt him to eat, but the most I achieved was an occasional dry biscuit or a small blancmange each morning. As the doctors came on their rounds I would express my concern that he was not eating. They seemed unconcerned and passed off my anxious questions with 'As long as he's taking fluids…' And so the weeks passed and the fluids were charted. But my baby, who could eat three square meals a day before he came to London, now flatly refused to eat at all. He should have been reweaned, of course.

It was ridiculous, I see now, to expect him to eat the same solid food after such massive haemorrhages. Toddler meals were brought and charted … 'refused'.

We were, I discovered, somewhat of an embarrassment to the hospital because of the publicity surrounding the transplant of Simon Bostic. This had caused complete disruption in the hospital and they wished to avoid a repetition. Mrs Elizabeth Bostic had two sons, apparently healthy and normal. Then Andrew, a toddler, was discovered to have granulomatous, a bone marrow disease. As Liz watched Andrew die a horrific death from septicaemia she was informed her baby, Simon, had the same disease. The only cure was a bone marrow transplant. Several successful ones had been performed at the Westminster Children's Hospital using a member of the family as donor.

Being a donor is a fairly simple and safe process. A small amount of marrow, a blood-like substance, is drawn from the hip bones or chest bones with a special needle under a general anaesthetic and the body soon replaces it. This healthy marrow is then dripped in the patient's bloodstream to recolonise the bones and reproduce itself, making healthy cells that the patient lacks. No member of Liz's family proved compatible and, learning that it was possible to find a donor from the public, Liz appealed in desperation for volunteers through a large national newspaper. Thousands of calls jammed the hospital's switchboard, not only at Westminster Hospital but hospitals, surgeries, and blood transfusion centres. It caused mayhem for the routine and emergency cases. As a mother I can fully appreciate her actions. I can also see that for the hospital it must have been a disaster. However, at the Cambridge Hospital, after testing just a handful of volunteer donors, a Cambridge housewife proved compatible with Simon. She donated some of her bone marrow and saved Simon's life. Between them they created a first in medicine. We followed in the wake of this disruption and sensational Press coverage.

Even if a close relative or friend phoned the hospital to ask about Anthony or to try to speak with me 'No comment' was the only reply they received.

I was warned not to speak with reporters or Mrs Bostic. Yet I did meet Mrs Bostic, a small intense woman with pretty blonde hair. 'Call me Liz, Shirley,' she said. 'I feel we know each other so well.' As we sat in my room in the mothers' unit, Liz related in detail the agony of losing Andrew and her struggle to save Simon. Her action required no justification to me. As a mother she did what she had to do. We vowed to keep in close contact.

One day, scanning the notes placed outside Anthony's room for the visiting senior paediatrician, I noted a letter from one doctor to another stating: 'We have another stinker on our hands.' I was furious, yet what could I do? Sadly I turned and looked at my once bright toddler, now listless and withdrawn. It was as if he was suspended in a time vacuum. Not eating, he was not growing or developing at all. And being completely shut away in this tiny room 12 ft by 10 ft – there were even metal grills on the windows as a safety measure – he was becoming more and more withdrawn. He no longer smiled or looked about him. Little wonder. He must have examined every square inch, every object in that room and the little he could see outside of it. He now just lay inert in his cot or preferred to curl, foetal position, in his pusher while I sang his favourite songs over and over again. Hour after hour each day I pushed him to and fro in the limited space. We were like trapped animals pacing our cage.

I could see the babies in the heart unit opposite and I vividly remember the new born babies rushed in and the sobbing parents through the glass barrier ... a silent movie live for my viewing. One baby died as the vicar prayed, just the two of them alone. I could envisage the mother, like myself at Anthony's birth, awaiting news of her baby. She had seen her baby only for a few moments and I saw it die before she even knew. The pusher rolled backwards and forwards as the tears welled and dropped silently, as lullabies for Anthony continued.

On another occasion a baby was being cared for by a nurse and went into cardiac arrest. The emergency buzzer rang. There wasn't time to pull the screens as the sister pounded the tiny chest and the doctor frantically tried mouth-to-mouth resuscitation. All in vain. The silent drama ended and the loss was shared. I bit my lip until the blood ran and pushed and sang, pushed and sang and thought each time that witnessing the death of a little one would become easier. But it doesn't, it doesn't. The death of a child is still an inexplicable enigma, a bud snapped ruthlessly from a tree before it has had a chance to bloom.

What a nightmare those long months must have been for my little son ... the monotony, the imprisonment, the handling by strange masked figures and the awakenings, to wonder if he would wake up at home *this* morning. I sang Anthony to sleep each night and climbed the two flights of stairs to the mothers' unit. I was not alone. One by one we would gather towards midnight. Those other mothers I remember so vividly; their love and courage were an inspiration. We would make tea on the little gas ring and gather to share our day. Some were in abject despair and grief, others cheered by the fact that their child could eat a little, had laughed, could breathe easier or was in less pain. We helped each other by just listening or proffering words of encouragement. Bound by our common battle to stay with our children at whatever cost, our emotions and bonds were analogous, in retrospect, to those of women in the war years. Not only did we daily fight along with our children in their struggle for life but we actually feared for their safety.

It was during the latter part of 1973 that London was ravaged by Irish Republican Army bombs. These vicious attacks would happen without notice. They were centred on the Westminster area because of its many government offices. One particularly savage bomb blasted Horseferry Road, next to Westminster Hospital. The building shook with the force of the explosion. Many people were seriously injured; one poor young woman lost her limbs. As one bomb after another illuminated the sky we prayed that our hospital would not be hit. What would happen to our children ... Anthony in isolation, others in highly inflammable oxygen tents, and those it would be a danger to move after delicate heart, brain, and spinal surgery?

Late one afternoon a bomb seriously damaged a building in Vincent Square, only a hundred yards away. One mother burst with hysteria and we rallied to calm her. She ran up and down the narrow corridor screaming; the strain of her existence and the menace of the bombs had caused her to snap. She had to leave us.

I seemed to lead a charmed existence, dodging attacks as if walking through a minefield and not stepping on a detonator. A short while before the Horseferry Road blast I had walked along the exact target area to the main hospital. In Vincent Square, seated on the steps of the soon-to-be-blasted building I had looked at the trees in their last golden blaze of autumn glory. The blaze that was to follow within the hour was less glorious.

I had been trying to come to terms with the apparent hopelessness of my situation. A few yards away, Anthony, in his cubicle, was having an afternoon nap. I could visualise his tiny, curled-up form, cheek resting on his hand and I thought, No, I will not give in! I will not turn back. This is where we are, this is where we stay, bombs and all.

The days and nights reverberated and echoed to an encore of sirens and ambulance wails, a parody of our inner mourning. Within a few days I missed several more bombs, one at Victoria Station, the nearest underground to the hospital, a second when we were evacuated at Tower Hill Underground and a third when the train strangely shot through Charing Cross, a major underground station, without stopping. Yet I cannot honestly say that I was afraid. The courage of the suffering children I had witnessed in the past years would have made fear of any kind a betrayal. I had that resigned feeling of 'what will be, will be.'

Yes, I did contemplate the horror of a bomb placed on an underground train packed with thousands of commuters and the Hades it would create in the bowels of the city. It was with great relief that I knew Anthony's cubicle was not facing onto the street as many victims had been brutally lacerated by flying glass. There were many hoax calls where hospitals and schools had to be evacuated. Streets were often blocked and trains stopped. It was chaos and probably worse than air-raids when at least there had been warning sirens and air-raid shelters. The people of London and other cities had, at the most, a few minutes' warning of the IRA bombs and sometimes none at all. Terrorism means just that. Strangely, despite the death toll and maimed bodies, people remained calm and the great pulsing heart of the city hardly missed a beat.

* * *

Apart from one mother I had been resident longest in the mothers' unit. Her daughter, eight years old, had leukaemia. She was a pale, elfin child, delicate and beautiful and I watched sadly each time she returned from chemotherapy treatment, grey and exhausted and weakening as the months dragged on. Lisa, the girl, was an only child. Her mother, Eileen, was a divorcee; intelligent and affluent. But the mothers' unit had no social or economic boundaries. One evening Eileen tapped at my door and entered. I could see she was distressed and utterly exhausted. She asked me how I felt about God.

'There is no God, Shirley, there can't be,' she said quietly. 'How can a God of love be ever present here within these walls, full of sick and dying children?' She told me that Lisa had almost died that night. Her hands encircled her cup of tea, as if she could obtain comfort from its warmth. 'I've tried to pray but it's no good, is it?' she went on. 'I honestly don't know, in my own heart,' I replied. 'I pray but I somehow feel unworthy to be heard. It's just that on two occasions I remember with such clarity – when Anthony was on the point of death – that I prayed and felt something. I can't explain it. I wish I could. All I know is that events followed so that Anthony did not die.'

'But Lisa knows she is dying,' Eileen sobbed. 'She's even requested to be cremated. She was quite calm, almost resigned, as if she didn't want to fight for her life anymore.' Our faces reflected our thoughts; a duplicate image of sorrow and incredulity as we sat now in silence. I had never really come to terms with death and nor had Lisa's mother. But a little girl had accepted the great mystery. Lisa died that night and I never saw Eileen again.

Marlene became a close friend. She had battled to keep her son, David, alive from birth for five years, to be strong enough to withstand delicate heart surgery. Her husband, Ray, travelled frequently from Devon to see them. David was saved and is now fit and well. We have corresponded since 1973. Soon after her return to Devon, Marlene wrote that Ray had cancer. Sadly he died and now she writes to me of her struggle as a widow and a nurse doing night duty to rear her family.

I write of these women with great admiration for their courage in battles that receive no glory or medals. These mothers, these unsung heroines ... Carol and her spina bifida daughter; Jean and her boy; Felicity with her two sons with hydrocephalus and Brenda with her little one, also spina bifida.

During an emergency they called Brenda to baptise her daughter and she exploded with anger, scattering the cloth and cross, screaming at the vicar that she didn't want that type of baptism as her daughter was not going to die. Neither did she.

This was the kind of guts and determination that brought their children through crises. Vividly I recollect the unselfish love and devotion and our night vigils to help each other through a special crisis.

Felicity was a schoolteacher, like myself, and we shared memories of our before-days and our joy in helping the healthy, fortunate ones at school. Her son Gregory survived but his little brother Charles died later of a brain tumour.

Unlike Brenda, Felicity had the help of her faith. She never wavered and was able to tell Gregory that his little brother had gone to Heaven and had been specially chosen to help there. But even now, when she phones me, Felicity says the ache of losing Charles is still there.

Each evening, one by one, we returned to the mothers' unit, discussed our children, our family, our hopes, our fears and our beliefs. There was grief, resignation, faith, bitterness, resentment – a vortex of emotions. We did not count the days. Rarely did we know which day of the week it was. We were there so long. Each glimmer of hope, each recovery, was a shared joy, each death a shared loss. Each knock on the door in the night set our hearts trembling. Which door? Whose child? I am sure each one of us was dreading the knock on *our* door.

Because we were there for so long the love and time needed for a sick child in the family meant a loss of the mother from the home. Other children in the family grieved and suffered, not having their mother at home with them. Husbands weakened, were unable to cope and deserted, often finding another woman for comfort. But how could a mother desert the sick child, the helpless one?

That unit gradually became our world, our family. The outside world seemed unreal. I occasionally left the hospital to shop for essentials but walking down a street, hearing the cacophony of traffic noise, I felt walled in glass. The people in Pimlico Market clustered around gay stalls, pulsating with life, colour and vendors' calls, and the normality of it all was too stark a contrast to our world just a few hundred yards away. I would stare at the harassed mums in the supermarkets, at the plump healthy toddlers in prams or tugging at their skirts and wonder if ever my little boy would be strong and free to join the world about us. I thought it would be a release to get out of the hospital environment for a while but it wasn't. It was as if I carried Anthony with me wherever I went as if the hospital was a huge shadow compelling me to return. One month merged into the next and still there was no further news of a potential donor. I was not then aware that the donor testing was slowly grinding to a halt.

* * *

In the late autumn I began to take Anthony out for walks around Vincent Square. Out of his isolation he was pale and listless and he remained always curled, foetal position, in his pusher hiding his eyes from the sunlight, as if the sky was too big for him. On those walks round and round the perimeter of the square, or within a fenced area on the grass, we were still prisoners pacing a larger compound. I tried to encourage Anthony to leave his pusher to walk, but he refused. He had withdrawn completely from the world.

I had time on those walks to wonder again if I had made the right decision in agreeing to prolong Anthony's life by the use of drugs. What had I achieved? It was as if each time I opened a door I walked smack into a brick wall. My guilt – yes, guilt – at being the cause of my son's suffering, purely and simply by wanting him and bearing him, made me sink to my knees on the grass beside his pushchair. I held him close and wished we could return to the beforetime when we were one and my heart beat for two; when he spiralled umbilical-held, balloon-soft, cushioned from the pain of this world.

* * *

Winter was approaching and I was advised that it would be better if I removed Anthony from the hospital environment because of the inevitable serious flu epidemics. I had already been trying to find us somewhere to live but all my friends in Britain had young children or pets (a potential source of infection). I asked for help from the welfare workers at the hospital. Their assistance was pathetic. I even asked if the church could help in some way. In all the seven months at Westminster Children's Hospital I was never once visited by a member of a church of any denomination.

I asked a member of the medical team if I could publicly appeal for suitable accommodation for Anthony so that he could be kept as infection-free as possible. It wasn't as if I was unwilling to pay rent, but as Anthony's restricted world revolved more and more around me it was difficult to leave him to flat hunt in London, a marathon task at the best of times. The reply was: 'No publicity' ... the ban still held. I recalled those words soon after when I decided to break that ban and fight again for Anthony's right to live. My girlfriend and ex-colleague, Frieda, found me an old Ford car for £35, so I set off to see what I could do. I drove as far north as Yorkshire where even the two-up, two-down Coronation Street-type of house was beyond our meagre resources. I tried caravan parks and searched from west to east, from Surrey to the edge of Kent. I drove hundreds of miles and for hours and hours each day.

I was nearing despair when I found a tiny, semi-derelict timber cottage in Thanet, Kent ... the cheapest of the agent's selection. It had been empty for a long, long time and the inner plaster board walls were bowed and damp. Two tiny rooms were downstairs and four upstairs. It even had a corrugated iron roof, not seen much in England, and a tiny square back yard and an outside loo. Raising the second mortgage on our home in Australia I bought it. Made of six-inch wide wooden slats once painted white, it propped against the post office on one side and half against the two next-door rickety timber cottages which supported each other like their aged occupants, two dear old ladies in their eighties. Their cottages were awaiting demolition while the land developers awaited their death. The ladies had refused rehousing. Having lived there all their lives, they wished to die in their humble homes which had been retainer cottages for the large neighbouring farmhouse and, before that, probably servant quarters or part of a coach house. A partly blocked side entrance allowed access to the back of the cottage which would have been wide enough for the passage of coaches or wagons. Behind, the flat fields stretched away to meet the sea at Pegwell Bay.

I went into nearby Ramsgate, a holiday resort with a colourful harbour of yachts and dinghies, as a stranger. I shopped for essentials: paper, paintbrushes, buckets, bowls, mops and disinfectant, beds and a cot for Anthony. The cottage already contained old carpets, curtains, a kitchen table, two chairs, an old gas fridge and a stove.

I returned to the hospital to care for Anthony. Dear mother, with directions written on a scrap of paper clutched bravely in her palm, caught a train to Ramsgate, a place she had never even heard of before, to find the cottage in the village of Manston. Single-handed she tackled the marathon job of scrubbing, cleaning, disinfecting and decorating No 8 to make a home for us and to enable us to leave the hospital.

Just a few days before Christmas at Pimlico Market I shopped with energy and interest for the first time since our arrival. I bought a bright silver Christmas tree and coloured electric lights; gay tinsel and trimmings and Christmas presents for Anthony and Mum. I loaded these and our suitcases into my battered little car, wrapped Anthony in a blanket, descended the hospital steps and handed him to Mum. Slamming my door and starting the engine was a herald to our freedom. At last we three had somewhere to go.

Almost sensing his escape Anthony was content to snuggle peacefully into his Nanna's lap and fell asleep to the lullaby of the windscreen wipers. His only reaction was to open his eyes each time the soothing motion stopped when the car halted at traffic lights or junctions. Perhaps, again, he was hoping he could wake up at home. But yet another strange place awaited this shattered little voyager.

Chapter 7

It was bitterly cold and raining as I headed out of London for Thanet, on the south-east coast of Kent. Anthony took little notice of the journey. The rain-blurred shops were gaily dressed for Christmas shoppers; Santa Claus and the reindeers bobbed and bright coloured lights on Christmas trees blinked. Leaving London behind, the wintry landscape sped past and the brown ploughed fields rolled away in folds on either side of the motorway, itself a bloodless incision on the landscape. The rain ceased on the approach to Thanet.

After leaving the M2 the road was a series of interminable roundabouts until, in the fading light, I sighted our last signpost and across the flat arable land the unmistakable markers of the cooling towers of the Pegwell Bay Power Station, standing like huge egg-timers, their bases swathed in the mist rolling in from the sea.

Anthony awoke as I parked in the narrow street by our front door, which entered directly on to the street. He gazed about him and resisted mother's attempts to take him out of the car. I took him from her, his puzzled face puckering to a howl of fear. I spoke quietly to him while mother unlocked the door and carried him into the cottage. It felt icy and damp as mother quietly lit the gas fires and drew the curtains on the grey Kent evening. We kept our outdoor clothes on while she unpacked the car and then made the indispensable, heartening cup of tea. Anthony didn't want to leave my arms, so I paced the floor, backwards and forwards, nursing him and singing to him for several hours. I was exhausted, mentally and physically, yet he clung to me until I felt we were moulded and were one again.

One of the upstairs rooms had a small gas fire and was now warm. Anthony had fallen asleep and I managed the steep stairs to place him in his cot, still clothed. I stared at his little face, pale with fatigue and so many months without sun and fresh air. I ached in every bone, yet my heart ached more for this little man who would awake to another strange new world. Later I sank thankfully into bed, and tucking my knees up to my chin, and with teeth chattering, sank into a deep sleep.

* * *

I awoke to Anthony's cry. Aching and stiff I lifted him from his cot in the bleak morning light. I noticed the damp patches in the corners of the bedroom walls and ceiling and felt the chill in my bones. I had kept the fires full on and prayed that I had done the right thing bringing him here.

We huddled round the gas fire in the small front room, Anthony climbing into his pushchair, conditioned to the habit; and while mother busied herself making this strange cottage home I sang Christmas songs to Anthony. I know he remembers this first Christmas as a toddler because 'Rudolf the Red-nosed Reindeer' is still his favourite Christmas song. That evening I decorated the Christmas tree and plugged in the Christmas lights, and my joy was a glimmer of a smile reflected in my baby's eyes. It rained interminably as if the skies were weeping for us.

We tried so hard to cheer each other, mother and I. On Christmas Eve I crossed the few yards to the village pub immediately opposite, appropriately named the Jolly Farmer and bought a bottle of sherry. I had bought the festive fare for Christmas Day, the small turkey, Christmas cake and Christmas pudding. We were expecting no guests, no visitors; we knew no one at all and my little son would not be eating a Christmas lunch.

After singing Anthony to sleep, I descended the stairs and joined Mum, seated in the soft glow of the Christmas tree lights. I studied their reflection in my glass of golden sherry. We wished each other a merry Christmas … this hard-to-break tradition even in the most bizarre of circumstances. But our eyes meeting reflected our concern for our little lad sleeping above, our loneliness this Christmas Eve, our sadness, our memories of the past two years and our fears for the future.

* * *

Christmas Day. We tried to be joyful for Anthony's sake, but all I could hear echoing in my ears were the words of the paediatrician: 'Children like Anthony rarely live beyond the age of two years.' I felt a wave of panic flood through me. Anthony had just passed his second birthday and this was his second Christmas; he was now living on borrowed time. It's a miracle he's alive at all, I thought. Why hadn't they found a donor for him? Why was this beautiful toddler playing on the floor with his Christmas toys dying, when he could be cured? Question after question in my head.

After our lunch alone mother and I took Anthony out of the cottage for his first outing. The apparently endless rain had at last ceased, leaving the sky in great folds of puffy grey. The street to the left meandered along, thinned to a muddy farm track and abruptly ended at a pig farm and a gate marked 'Keep Out: Ministry Property.' It barred entry to Manston Airfield. Turning back through the village – the pub on our left, our cottage and the village post office and only shop on our right – we crossed the road leading to the air terminal and discovered miles of flat arable land veined by numerous country lanes.

This first excursion produced no reaction from Anthony, who tucked his cold nose into his coat and, with only his bobble cap showing, slumped into his pusher. I was elated with what I had seen despite the gloomy grey and brown of it all. If only I could draw Anthony from his pusher, teach him to walk again … there were country lanes galore and sea air blowing across this peninsula, this isle of Thanet, which should put the glow back into his cheeks. The cottage appeared almost welcoming when we returned. That night we went to bed with more cheer and optimism since our arrival in England but it was short-lived. We were disturbed by Anthony's hacking cough and by morning he was feverish. I alerted the hospital and at first light I headed back to London. Exhausted by his persistent cough, Anthony appeared soothed by the drone of the car's engine and fell asleep in mother's arms. As I stopped outside the hospital he stirred, a look of expectation on his tired little face. Perhaps again, he thought he had made the journey back to his home in Australia and his nightmare was over. I went around to the passenger seat, taking him from mother and once more climbed the steps into the hospital.

Anthony reacted immediately; wide awake, he stared about him and recognising his surroundings, screamed in terror and struggled in my arms. I had to hold him tightly to restrain him, to manage the distance back to his isolation cubicle. Feeling near to tears myself and once again calling upon my reserves of self-control, calmly I crooned to him while the preliminaries were attended to ... temperature, pulse, blood tests, and chest examinations. He clung to me like a koala; his tear-smeared face, tired and puffy, lolled on my shoulder and his little punctured arm embraced my neck. It was late into the night before he slept in my arms and I was able to place him in his cot, quietly lock the side and bent with fatigue and sadness, slowly take the familiar route to my bed in the mothers' unit.

Even then I was to find an old friend standing also pale and tired by the gas ring, making tea, having been called in the night for yet another crisis with her little one.

Anthony had a chest infection and this period of hospitalisation enabled me to contact the gas company and have extra fires fitted in our cottage and the roof tiled to make it watertight. It was only apparent after such measures just how damp the cottage had been. Gradually, over the next few days, the bows in the walls levelled and the stains on walls and ceilings dried out and disappeared.

During this period in London I met Dr David James, Director of the Blood Transfusion Service and consultant pathologist to the main Westminster Hospital. I discovered he was responsible for the donor testing programme for bone marrow transplants ... a quietly spoken Welshman, small in stature. It was our first encounter and I was not immediately aware of his brilliance, vision and determination. I expressed my concern that no further donor had been found for Anthony since the American and was informed by Dr James that at this stage the testing of volunteer donors had come to a halt because of lack of funds. The one technician initially supported by a grant for this and other projects in the laboratory had left. The Ministry of Health had been approached but had refused to finance a replacement, so the testing could not continue. They had set up a working party to 'look into the situation'.

'We have thousands of willing volunteers,' said Dr James.

'But we now have no means of tissue-typing them. This involves taking a blood sample from each donor and examining it very carefully on special slides under a microscope; it is complex and time-consuming. We need to identify and code all the blood cells, not simply find a blood group. One laboratory technician working full time on donor-testing can tissue-type only five people a day.

'You know, Mrs Nolan, that Anthony's tissue-typing is exceptionally rare. Most patient's chances of compatibility are put at one in 10,000. Anthony's work out at somewhere near one in 50,000 which means we could test five donors and have his Mr Right turn up or have to plough through to 50,000.

'What I would like to see is a donor register compiled so that when a patient needs a donor, the information is immediately available. The need for this will become more and more urgent as advances are made in the treatment of bone marrow diseases and leukaemia and allied diseases. However, even with a technician working full time on this project it would take decades to compile such a register,' said Dr James.

Decades, I felt like screaming: But Anthony doesn't have decades! He may have only days. At this moment he's again fighting for his life. 'Simon Bostic was lucky,' continued Dr James. 'A colleague of mine co-operated despite the problems of publicity and his donor was found in the first batch tested in Cambridge.

I must add that other hospitals and blood transfusion centres have said they cannot spare staff to tissue type volunteers in their areas because of the heavy workloads for routine work.'

Somehow, I was listening, digesting all that this kind Welshman was saying, and on the surface it appeared to mean that nothing more could be done. But I sensed Dr James did not feel this way ... he wanted to continue this work.

My mind had weighed the information like a computer and out came the question: 'How much would it cost to pay the salary of a laboratory technician?'

'In the region of £3,000 a year,' replied Dr James, a gleam in his eye.

'All right, I will find that £3,000,' I said. Here was a man who believed something could be done; so did I. I hadn't given in by a long shot. I didn't know how on earth I would get £3,000 but I knew I had to. I thought of the millions wasted by governments, and here I was trying to think of ways to raise £3,000 to save children's lives. It didn't make sense. I would laugh if it wasn't all so bloody tragic!

In the Australian media at the same time was corresponding criticism of Labour Prime Minister Gough Whitlam's personal expenditure whims, which infuriated the Australian taxpayer and, among other things, eventually ousted him from power. The irony is that both governments to whom I appealed then were Labour governments with policies which expound the rights of the underprivileged. It appears, like George Orwell's Animal Farm, that our leaders were sidetracked somewhere along the line ... All men are equal but some are more equal than others. Even now, as I write this, politicians everywhere are under fire for megalomania style spending of millions upon millions on the purchase of jets for personal use, yet hundreds of thousands of people are unemployed.

There is despair, poverty, yet children who can be cured are blatantly allowed to die.

At the hospital with Anthony, each newspaper article highlighting wastage of public monies infuriated me. I paced my bedroom in the mothers' unit, smashing my fists at the walls; I was supposed to accept that there was no money to save my son; his life was not important. But what could I do, having to care for a little boy so critically ill?

* * *

In late January, Anthony was able to return to the cottage. I made a determined effort to stimulate him as much as possible, playing nursery rhymes and children's songs. I worked again on his weakened leg muscles, encouraging him to jump and dance, and I persisted in taking him out daily down the country lanes into the fresh air. While he huddled in his push chair I was muttering to myself, how are you going to get £3,000?

The village post office shop was the nerve centre of the village by day and the Jolly Farmer pub took over at night. I came to know the owners, Peter and his wife, very well. After all, two of my upstairs rooms were directly over his shop and each thump of a stamp on a postal order and each clang of the till registered above and below. The post box was an insertion into a neck in our front room. Peter was, so-to-speak, the eyes and ears of the village. He knew everyone and all gossip was aired between the loaves of bread on one side and the tins of fruit on the other. Anything of interest he relayed to the local newspaper. Of course, I spoke to him of Anthony, of Australia and now of our desperate plight. And that evening a young reporter, Graham Sutherland from the *Kentish Express,* knocked at No 8 High Street, Manston.

I had no fears now of breaking the publicity ban. Anthony's life was at stake. I could no longer remain silent. Anthony could not be treated without a donor and all testing had stopped. I welcomed this reporter and told him my story from the beginning. I did, however, explain what had happened previously when Liz Bostic's story about Simon was publicised and asked that people not ring the hospital. A front-page story appeared the next day in the *Kentish Express* and the village was on red alert for the first time since the war years, when Manston Airfield was the nearest to Europe. At the post office, the pub, the garage, every phone in the village was ringing in unison with wonderful people misinterpreting the story and thinking we needed a blood donor. To prevent opening the door so many times and disturbing Anthony and subjecting him to the cold I stood out in the street and greeted the convoys of cars with prepared slips of paper stating, 'please send your name and address and age to Dr James, Westminster Hospital. Please write, do not phone.' The first man to arrive was the mechanic from the Manston garage, still clad in his overalls. He had literally downed tools and, producing his blood donor card, offered to help Anthony.

This wonderful, spontaneous reaction was one of thousands. Even if it involved pain, discomfort, self-funding, time off work, or whatever cost, not knowing what was involved, people stepped forward to volunteer to save Anthony's life ... Incredibly, even if it meant sacrificing their own life.

* * *

After a feature in the national Press one experience made me humbly weep. A knock at my door revealed a smartly dressed elderly gentleman. As we allowed no one into the cottage all filming and interviews were done outside to protect Anthony from infection and contact with others. I asked the old chap to come through the side passage to the back yard. This man, in his 70s, had driven hundreds of miles from Wales – the width of England – to offer his actual body, his life, if it could be used, to save Anthony. He said he was a widower, had led a good life and would deem it a fulfilling end to give a child the chance to do the same. Such a drive in Britain, with its busy roads, towns and cities, would have taken this old gentleman all day, yet I could not even welcome him into my home. How do you tell someone who has made such a gesture that it is not needed, that he was even too old to be a bone marrow donor? I couldn't. I thanked him over and over again, brought hot tea to drink outside and listened to a part of his now lonely life.

The *Kentish Express* was besieged by volunteers, and so the frontpage story continued. Confusion reigned. Before Anthony's diagnosis I had never heard of bone marrow disease, either. Like most people I thought of bone marrow as good for stews or feeding to dogs. The southern TV news programme, 'Day by Day', covered the story, which triggered off more volunteers. The TV people kindly directed mail to me and I replied to each inquiry with person: 21 handwritten letters, coping with the mail late in the evening, when Anthony was finally asleep. At that time I couldn't type, nor did I possess a typewriter. The cost of phone calls, stamps and stationery I funded personally. Gradually, piece by piece, the story unfolded and the wonderful people of Thanet had an aim to raise the £3,000. for that technician. The Mayors of Thanet, Ramsgate, Margate and Broadstairs joined to support me. I owe our start mainly to those town councillors and to the local Midland Bank Manager, Mr Hearn, who acted as honorary treasurer.

The people set about organising their raffles, coffee mornings, jumble sales and sponsored events, but it took time; and time was the least factor in Anthony's favour. But it was heartening to feel the spirit of this community pulling with me, feeling that one little boy was worth saving. The Mayoral office in Margate printed some single leaflets, and while Anthony had his midday nap and mother cared for him, I delivered one to every pub, shop and factory in the area and explained at length to those who would listen about this 'bone marrow thing'. Pfizer, the drug company at nearby Sandwich, understood. I battled my way through the secretaries to the under-manager and the manager and explained about the compiling of our donor register. They donated £500, our first major donation.

On and on I drove, day after day, and walked all over Thanet. Everywhere I went the streets were ablaze with orange posters: DYING BABY APPEAL. I gritted my teeth, hunched my shoulders and muttered: 'That's my baby and he's NOT going to die.' Fortunately the national Press continued the local story, the original publicity of Simon and Anthony was recalled, and at last the story was told in full. In both Britain and Australia the reporters did all they could to help. Alan Hargreaves, of Thames Television, came to the cottage and 1974 heralded the first TV documentary of Anthony's plight.

In the early summer of 1974 came the tremendous news that Kamahl, the wonderful entertainer in Australia, had personally donated £3,000. A cheque presentation by representatives of the Save the Children Fund in London to Dr James was arranged. The first technician was able to be trained to restart testing, and by the end of 1974, with the money raised by the people of Thanet and a corresponding appeal by the Adelaide Advertiser in Australia, a second technician joined our team.

Our days were full. Besides delivering leaflets and attending local committee meetings and then others with Dr James at Westminster, talking to the many reporters – both local, national, and international – conducting radio and TV interviews and answering mail, I had the main task of keeping Anthony alive and trying to undo some of the drastic side effects of his long isolation.

After his morning walk he was usually back for a nap by 10 or 11 a.m. I would then set off campaigning while Mum looked after him, cleaned the cottage and prepared lunch. I would have dearly loved to try to rest also, but if Anthony was to have any hope of life I must tell people about his struggle, and other children like him.

We spent our evenings playing in our limited space. Anthony's favourite game was walking up and down the two steep flights of stairs in the cottage. I guarded him carefully but encouraged him because the exercise helped to strengthen his legs; or we played in the bathroom, floating matches and sliding them down the bath's sides, creating a miniature logging lake. My bed was a tempting play area as we rollicked and I tickled him, indulging in the usual horseplay that kids adore. I also taught him to bounce, holding my hands out, using the bed as a trampoline. I can still see those little legs moving as pistons, up and down, and hear Anthony's chuckles. But most of all, incredibly, he grew stronger and sturdier. Gradually, like spring flowers on those daily walks, he began to unfurl and sit up and look about him.

* * *

I was aware that in the cottage he showed no interest in his surroundings. He never even looked at the gay pictures I had pasted on his bedroom wall. It was as if he assumed he was still in his hospital room. He'd examined it so many times, itemised it all and ceased to look. Because he was programmed again at temperature times to wake frequently our nights were restless and tiring. Many nights he would awake crying and we would comfort him, reassuring him that it was a nightmare and we were all here together. Mother and I took it in turns to do the first shift, as we called it. It was not uncommon to be playing games or singing nursery rhymes at 4.30 a.m. We were always awake long before the bakery and milk deliveries to the post office below. Those winter and spring mornings it seemed an eternity before dawn broke; somehow it was less wearying when it was daylight.

With Anthony waking so early we were out at the crack of dawn. The air was fresh and the sun came up out of the sea, tinting the lanes and tracks. I took him into the playground of a local home for deserted children or those from problem homes. The children knew us from the newspapers and would willingly come and say hello. They never came too near Anthony because of the infection risk but they would call and show him their favourite toys; and slowly he began to respond. One bright spring morning after an early shower the children from the council home were careering, chortling and splashing in and out of large, muddy puddles. Anthony sat and watched and then hesitantly tried to stand up in his push chair. So I lifted him out. Taking my hand, poised like a gosling in his little red wellingtons, he launched into the first puddle. Backwards and forwards he went. He firmly clutched my hand for support. Splish! Splosh! He kicked and parted the muddy puddles. I was soaked and mud-spattered and so was he, but we didn't care and the children cheered. This was his first reaction to the outside world since leaving Australia. Mother went into Ramsgate and bought Anthony some fisherman's pants. They were far too big so she cut them down and elasticised the bottoms, and we fitted them over his pants and Wellington tops. Mum and I rigged out in knee-length farmer's rubber boots made an elegant sight any Kent morning, tramping each muddy section of those country lanes ... Lowry figures, two long, one short, in a winter's landscape.

Eagerly now Anthony clambered into his pushchair and, once out of the village, it was left abandoned and this tiny tot literally walked miles. It was usually returned home for us or left untouched. It was distinctly Anthony's, covered with multi-coloured flowers and stamped in bold letters 'Made in Australia'.

We became a familiar sight, puddle-jumping, and no longer got raised eyebrows but instead a friendly wave or greeting. Many a weary British or Australian camera crew have been outdistanced or frozen into submission by my intrepid traveller, exalting in his freedom, cheeks fiery red, striding out with the gait of a sturdy Shetland pony as he explored his new world.

* * *

Our struggle for Anthony's life became a symbol of the fight for the rights of the individual in a society where only the rich, the notorious, the politicians or unions – those groups epitomising the big, the powerful – appeared to have a voice. This was reflected in the thousands of letters I received giving encouragement, and the continuous support of the media who expressed admiration that I would not give in ... I would not take no for an answer ... that I believed one little child and all he represented was worth fighting for. These same people also wrote to the British Prime Minister and to Barbara Castle, Minister of Health. And they received replies to the effect that not enough research had been completed to warrant a funding of the project. However, when we approached well-known companies and trusts for a research grant – such as the Nuffield Foundation and Wellcome Trust – we were told that tissue-typing was routine medical technique and did not qualify for a research grant. That's what I call having a ball in neither court. Later replies were to infuriate me even more. I would sit in my tiny back kitchen literally gnashing my teeth, spitting imprecations. One letter from Barbara Castle's department was to the effect that the problem was one of lack of testing sera and not of money, as this project was being supported by charity. Bloody cheek, I thought. Me, I was that charity, sitting, pen poised to answer the piles of letters from the public that would take me well into the night. Any concerned lay members of the public who received such a reply would either assume that money was not needed (yet here was I trying desperately to raise money to pay the salaries of laboratory technicians so that testing could continue) or that everything possible was being done and the hold-up was not the responsibility of the Department of Health. It was a shortage of testing sera!

How was the public to even know what testing sera was! It could have been rhino's cells from Africa as far as they were concerned. And so the letters poured out from the Department of Health, coolly, effectively extinguishing the fires of the articulate who were asking for an explanation and receiving the usual bureaucratic half-truths. My local MP, Jonathan Aitken, tried to raise the issue in the House of Commons and could do no more than return with the reply that the situation was being 'looked into'. Who was doing the looking and at what they were looking we never did find out. The facts were clear enough but then politicians never could see the obvious solution to a problem. A donor register was needed. Children – and adults – like Anthony, without a relative to donate bone marrow, needed a compatible donor from the public. The public had shown their willingness to participate by volunteering in their thousands. All that was needed was the means to take, test and code the blood samples. It was as simple as that. A working party was set up but we never discovered who it comprised and it was blatantly obvious that the funding of such a working party would have paid for the project's completion many times over.

I soon learned that, at this stage, venting my frustration and anger towards the government or a government department was producing negative results and only draining my depleted and much-needed energy. Perusing letters and press statements, it was obvious that the corridors of power are really mirrored mazes, each door a reflected reflection. Each so-called public servant from the Prime Minister down passes the proverbial buck down one tier of the public service ladder. Each little servant is not responsible. His current superior is, right up to the Minister of Health, who passes it to the Prime Minister, who passes it back to the Department of Health. And so the slow-motion relay continues and the bureaucratic roundabout happily revolves. The support from the public was my mainstay when spirits flagged. They did not give in but continued to demonstrate their belief in the rights of the individual by positive action. Spreading slowly over the whole country was a tide of goodwill as people related to a little boy called Anthony Nolan. In villages, towns and cities people gathered in whatever way they were able to organise fundraising activities.

Our project was indebted especially to the Round Table organisation, a community aid group. I was asked to speak to the Broadstairs Tablers, an exclusively male domain. I was the first female guest speaker allowed in their midst for eight years. I faced this distinguished gathering and carefully – and simply – explained the basics of our medical project. Two of the members were biochemists, George Hawkes and Alan Smith, who worked at a large local laboratory breeding a special kind of white rat for medical research. They understood, possibly better than I, the technicalities of tissue-typing, and its complexity and value.

From that gathering of Tablers they voted to support us. They circulated information to Round Tablers throughout Britain, asking for their support. The Broadstairs Round Table alone raised more than £20,000 but, more than that, they were the catalyst, triggering a chain reaction of other forms of help, equally valuable as donations or fundraising activities. The Round Table organisation consists mainly of businessmen and includes doctors, dentists, scientists and the like. Many of their wives are members of the Ladies Circle, the feminine equivalent of the Round Table. Some of these ladies were also medically qualified to assist our work. Under the direction of Dr James at Westminster they volunteered to hold donor bleeding sessions. Using their local paper and their own resources, they advertised when a donor session would operate in their area. Dr James and our technicians would arrange the dispatching of empty blood syringes and donor forms. Each evening the Tablers and their wives would not only make their premises available for the donors but would man telephones, organise the numbers to correlate with the number the technicians would test, take the blood samples, label and pack the syringes, complete the donor forms and ensure the safe delivery of the batches so they were awaiting the technicians each morning in the laboratory.

The first area session of this kind was held in Buckinghamshire and ran for several months, providing the technicians with a regular supply. This was greatly aided by a kind lady, Mrs Marion Matthews, a journalist who gave marathon support, fundraising locally and on a larger scale.

It was impossible to qualify the value of this system, which is still in use today, as one Round Table takes over from another, from Crowborough, Gravesend, Eastbourne, Brighton and so on. It saves hard-pressed staff from having to take blood samples from donors or wait for donors to find their way to a busy hospital in the centre of London. It means. they are free to begin work immediately each morning. But what is more important is that it enables the programme to function more efficiently and speedily.

One technician can test approximately five samples a day. With two technicians working full time we were able to test 40 to 50 volunteers a week. I still felt we were not working speedily enough to save Anthony, but at least each week he had a one-in-fifty chance. It was a longshot with his odds of compatibility as great as one in 50,000. I told myself that Anthony was still alive and testing had restarted. Now my task was two-fold: to keep Anthony alive until his donor was found and to ensure that testing continued and, if possible, to employ more technicians to swell the numbers tested.

I could think of nothing else. My life was now dedicated to this end. It solely revolved around Anthony and the Appeal. When I spoke to Dr James about the donor register and my desire to try to raise more money to pay more technicians he fully understood my urgency and desperation. But he had to explain: 'I'm afraid the two technicians working on this project are housed in already cramped laboratories in my department. We simply don't have any space for more.' But I pressed on and raised more money and wonderful Dr James did squeeze four technicians somehow into that labyrinth of tiny labs in the basement of Westminster Hospital. This was made possible by the continued support of the Press and the public of Britain and Australia.

A local reporter, Neville Nisse, and his lovely wife, Shula, worked hard and arranged three successful variety shows in the seaside resorts of Ramsgate and Margate. Top British stars gave their services free. John Mills, Roy Castle, Roy Hudd, Max Wall, Ann Shelton, Roger de Courcey, Charles Smithers, Frank Finlay (from the moving TV series 'Bouquet of Barbed Wire'); Bruce Forsythe even did a one-man show for the Appeal. All these highly paid entertainers stopped in their world of glitter and glory and thought of one small boy and what he stood for. I shall always remember them with gratitude and warmth. I was able to meet many of these stars and thank them personally. This is my sincere public thanks to them. I met Bruce Forsythe before his performance. He is as vibrant and humorous off-stage as on. Similarly, I met Frank Finlay, acting as compere for Neville's third show. As we sat in his dressing room I was impressed by his overpowering gentleness, warmth, and genuine modesty when he expressed nervousness at compering the show.

'I've never done anything like this before,' he said. I laughed and said, 'Neither had I until a few months ago.' He was wonderful. They were all wonderful.

Chapter 8

Anthony had remission periods but plagued by constant urinary tract infections, would lapse into critical haemorrhaging phases. During one period of several months he was supported constantly by antibiotics as well as steroids. Again, the night-time sniffles, the streams of blood everywhere, the hours of trying to calm my terrified little boy. Again, again and again. I became an expert at preparing myself for bleeding sessions. Anthony's eyes became puffy, sometimes mere slits, the pupils an opaque dark grey, the bridge of his nose appeared blue, the skin like tissue paper. Within hours the blood flowed.

We spent hours thinking over ways we could protect Anthony even more. Mother said we should sterilise everything he used and give him boiled water. I decided the cottage needed to be cleaner. Gradually we adapted the cottage to deal with Anthony's complex illness. Inside and out we ensured it was as aseptic and as safe as possible. I concreted the backyard, doing the mixing with bucket and shovel. The first day was the hardest until my arm and back muscles toned to the work. I smoothed the finished work with the fat of my palms to leave the finish even enough to ensure Anthony would not trip. He fell and bruised easily.

When the north-east winds blew off the sea he could still toddle out and play. The high-fenced backyard was protected and a suntrap. During the summer months he could romp completely naked and splash about in his inflatable wading pool, and we were able to welcome the occasional visitor who could trek the long journey to our cottage. When possible my brother Tony came or my cousin Linda. Anthony enjoyed their play and attention. These were happy times as we cavorted in our tiny backyard. We were as brown as anything.

While mother was playing with Anthony I had turned my hand from concreting to painting the exterior of the house. The timber, dingy and peeling, was unsightly. I set to work using a ladder from the post office to repaint it a brilliant white with the doors and window frames a contrasting black. The heavy ladder on my shoulder, heaving to and fro, I only needed a bowler hat to qualify for a replica of a figure in a Charlie Chaplin movie.

We replaced the original old carpets with the vinyl floor covering to ensure the rooms could be mopped and disinfected daily and kept dust free. Anthony is allergic to dust. It activates his eczema. Mother painted the interior walls white so they, too, could be wiped or, after heavy haemorrhaging, be re-painted. The really distressing times were when Anthony appeared to have a migraine attack. He would bash his head on the walls and furniture, leaving a trail of bloody smears and hand marks. He was duly fascinated and terrified by the ghastly red patterns left on his hands, wiped across his face, and the slaughterhouse streaks left by his face, wiped across the white walls. When the bleeding stopped the cottage looked like a scene of brutal butchery.

As in Australia, these haemorrhages invariably happened in the dark hours before dawn and the procedure was the same ... backbreaking hours of nursing; mother changing and soaking bloodied swab after swab. We three were living the same drama over and over. The actors were the same. Only the scenes were changed. A different town, a different country and a different hospital on standby.

Our measures worked to a degree. Although Anthony still haemorrhaged, the urinary tract infections disappeared and he no longer needed antibiotics. He continued, however, on the steroid drugs. No one directed me otherwise. This made his body disproportionate. He had a large, round, chubby face and a shortened body with tiny legs. But my ignorance, and perhaps the difficulty facing the doctors dealing with such a rare disease, meant that we accepted this drug as his lifeline. Today my six-and-a-half-year-old son, as I write this, is barely a few inches taller, or a kilo or two heavier, than those days in Manston four years ago. It is as if his condition, or this drug, have anchored him in time, a toddler forever.

Our life followed a pattern, as most lives do. But instead of waves of normality or excitement, it was measured by how many bleeds Anthony had each month, how many interviews were planned, how many fundraising events I could attend, and how many lectures I could give. We worked as a team, mother and I. I cared for Anthony, treated his skin and haemorrhages, tried to feed him, took him for walks, taught him, while mother kept the house spic and span, prepared our meals and cared for Anthony when I had to go out. One of us was always with him. We never went out socially in all those months, in hospital and at Manston. The only time my dear mother left Anthony was to attend her father's funeral in a small mining town in Yorkshire in the north of England. She was bowed with grief. She had been unable to visit grandfather in his last days because of the infection risk to Anthony.

If I accepted an engagement I planned it to coincide with Anthony's nap or bedtimes, so I left him as little as possible. TV interviews were still conducted outside and radio interviews were by telephone or recorder, until I learned to use the BBC's small broadcasting centre at nearby Canterbury, where I would let myself in, link up with London and broadcast live. We still allowed no one to enter the cottage or to be in close contact with Anthony. Outside he could be filmed without contact and even enjoyed the film crews and the cameras. He could see the villagers going about their day and be greeted by them, but he always headed for the children's home. It was heartbreaking to see him want to play with and touch the children, who instinctively moved out of his reach. On reflection, how rejected, how bewildered Anthony must have been. His instinctive reaching out for other human contact inevitably resulted in the object of his attention visibly avoiding him, stepping away from him. It was difficult to keep friendly cats and dogs at bay, as they were also a potential infection risk. Dogs jump up and lick faces. I had to shoo them away and soon, conditioned at the sight of a pet, Anthony piped in with, 'Shoo, dog, shoo, pussy,' and crossed the road away from them. I tried to keep the 'don'ts' as limited as possible but normal, healthy children like to be messy, to touch, to pick up and collect objects nauseating to adults.

Somehow, I had to try to undo the damage of isolation and still let Anthony behave as normally as possible. As Anthony relaxed and came to know his new world he was as mischievous, as curious as any other toddler. He spotted a horse one day way over in a distant paddock. I could see no lane or footpath but, undeterred, Anthony dragged me diagonally across a wet ploughed field to examine the object of his attention who, condescendingly, whinnied a greeting, much to Anthony's delight. We examined barns, richly aromatic with stored seed potatoes, row upon row like a vertical garden, and played hide and seek between the stacked boxes, the stretched sun's rays filtering through the barn's slats, tinting the scene shades of earthy brown. We examined rusted plough shares, crawled under discarded wagons of bygone days and swung on their shafts. In a moment of quiet I could see the sturdy horse pawing the ground, his twitching nostrils steaming in the cold of dawn, edging to begin the day's work, and the jocular villagers huddled together on the cart to keep warm.

As we explored the area, its ploughed fields richly textured in Van Gogh swathes, the scene was little changed from years past. The rich arable land yielded three or four rotated crops a year. Only now the lanes buzzed with tractors instead of hoofbeats. Already out and about, Anthony and I greeted the fine, sturdy, scarved field workers, women wrapped up in protective layers of clothing as if they were scarecrows, bundled on the back of farm wagons, heading for the cabbages or potatoes, singing cheerily, the songmaster a ruddy-faced farmer proudly perched up front steering his load into the dawn. We would return red-cheeked and glowing and Mum would help peel off our muddy gum boots, pants, caps, scarves, coats and mittens.

I was ravenous, but I could never coax Anthony to eat. I tried all kinds of food. Baby rice, tasty broths, fruits, offering small amounts, trying to coax him to sip even a teaspoonful, all to no avail. Each meal mother prepared I handed Anthony a fork or a spoon and sat him on my lap. He sniffed at the food appreciatively then, happily spearing a sprout, carrot or other forkable pieces thrust them into my mouth.

I prepared his usual chocolate mousse-type food and from the local health food shop added high protein supplement, a powder which dissolved easily into the milk. The chocolate camouflaged the mild, nutty flavour. This, vitamin drops and pure blackcurrant juice, was all he would accept. Unhappily I tried several times to wrap him cocoon-fashion in a large, soft towel and make him take a spoonful of broth. He would spit it out and the struggle would precipitate a nosebleed, so I desisted.

I realised that Anthony had not grown at all in the eight months since we had left Australia. I was fully aware of what constituted a properly balanced diet. He was suffering from malnutrition. I just couldn't understand how my previously ravenous one-and-a-half-year-old was now totally disinterested in food. Gradually, as mother served a meal, I couldn't touch it. I sat with Anthony and swallowed without tasting the pieces which he fed to me. But I no longer enjoyed food. How could I eat when Anthony was starving himself?

It was only years later, on our return to Australia, that psychiatric study of Anthony confirmed my theory – a journey of 12,000 miles, a massive internal haemorrhaging resulting in him bleeding his bowel lining, and the trauma of seven months' hospital isolation, had such a profound effect that Anthony associated food with this· unhappy period.

I continued offering all foods and, to my surprise, one morning Anthony accepted Weetabix and milk. I used honey instead of sugar to sweeten it. This diet, similarly repetitious; replaced the chocolate mousse, but at least it was a nutritious change.

The months had passed, bringing with them the warmth of summer. The Appeal was gathering momentum. At two-and-a-half Anthony was still alive. More letters were arriving from all over the world, bringing words of encouragement and expressing concern for Anthony. They strengthened my determination to fight on. We three were not alone any longer. People everywhere – friends, yet strangers to us – were willing Anthony to live. We were enveloped in a mysterious web of goodwill, spun as the world revolved.

That summer we received two rather special visitors, Kamahl and his lovely wife Sohodra. While on tour in England they came to our little cottage to see Anthony, bringing a huge talking teddy almost as big as Anthony himself. They, too, cared about one little boy's battle to live.

Kamahl left several of his record albums, and his song 'I'll Give You A Daisy A Day' became Anthony's favourite. Our pocket handkerchief backyard was a jostle of photographers as Anthony happily sat on Kamahl's lap; he wasn't playing with the teddy – but Sohodra's beautiful pearls, which he had deftly removed and now held him fascinated as they reflected the sun.

I was incredulous when I received a phone call one day telling me that Coco, the world's most famous clown, had heard of Anthony and his lonely life. Anthony could not go to the circus so Coco would bring the circus to him. To a fanfare of trumpets and the bang of drums the mini-circus turned into the village and from the first gaily painted wagon appeared Coco the Clown. Villagers, their children and an entourage of Press and TV cameras pressed forward. We greeted this most remarkable of clowns, Anthony cradled in my arms, fascinated by such a gathering, as the cameras whirred and flash after flash exploded. the mask of white on Coco's face was a patchwork of colour; blue and orange crescents around the eyes and criss-crossed with black bars. The mouth, exaggerated, was garish red and swelled to a fixed grin. Perhaps only I saw the kind but tired smile beneath the grease paint, the veined gentle old eyes, watery and rainbow-reflected by their coloured rims.

My eyes glistened as I held the frail hand, its skin folded like fine parchment, the ridged veins dotted with brown age spots. Our eyes held, we understood. We were on show and we each had to play our part. Coco triggered applause by pulling a hidden cord somewhere in his floppy patchwork suit which made his bright henna wig rise in the air and return to his bald head. The children cheered as Coco flapped his clown-size shoes over to a second wagon to reveal a baby elephant. The circus handlers had set out a circular stand on which the elephant climbed, then pivoted to the music from the band. The scene was played out as Coco circled like the elephant to the music, cheers and hand-clapping. Yet all I could see was a dear old man beneath it all, the bowed shoulders and the carefully manoeuvred gestures. I wanted to weep with gratitude, no, something much deeper, for this greatest of performers who was staging his final performance for the love of Anthony. In his 80s, Coco died just a few weeks later.

I charted carefully Anthony's drugs and haemorrhages. He had now gone a month without a setback. I stared happily at my blank chart on the pantry wall, standing beside the months which I marked off. If the present occupants of No. 8 High Street, Manston, examine the wall in the pantry carefully they will see the months we lived there faithfully marked, just as I had done in my pantry in Australia. I always marked six months in advance. It was a challenge to me to bring Anthony through that period alive. Despite the eating problem he had learned to walk again. He was chatting like a magpie and managing without blood transfusions. I thought him the cutest little fellow in Christendom.

As I watched him develop the sharp edges of his suffering rounded and melted a little. I was overjoyed that he could see, walk, hear and talk. A child's first words – not just the 'Mumma' and 'Dadda' kind – but the understanding words are a great joy. We could communicate. I began to relax in the warmth of our new rapport. Those early morning hours before the dawn I now earnestly taught

Anthony as well as played with him. He was not a vegetable. He learned quickly and remembered everything.

Until one morning he did not herald the dawn. I was programmed to wake early and thought Anthony was sleeping unusually well, but a mother's intuition made me peep into the nursery. I found him feverish and bloodsoaked in his cot. I called in our local GP who expressed the view that Anthony had measles. If this was so I knew he could die within 48 hours. Back again to Westminster Hospital! Anthony was rigid with terror. Thank God, he did not have measles, only the recurring urinary infection. But it still took me several weeks to undo his regression. Night after night he awoke sobbing from a nightmare and mother or I would sit with him through the night hours to comfort him.

When we left Adelaide we had expected to be gone no longer than six months. This had now stretched into almost a year, and I missed Ted. He had written frequently and I had made tape recordings for him of my thoughts and feelings and, later especially, of Anthony's first words, phrases and attempts to sing. I didn't want him to miss any of Anthony's toddler development. Now the day was almost here and he would arrive from Australia to visit us. My first thoughts were whether Anthony would recognise his father, what I would say at the airport, if he thought I had changed. The past year had been tough. I had lost weight and as I looked at my work-roughened hands I thought of the manicured ones that once accompanied me to school.

We spotted each other instantly. Ted appeared through the Customs gate and without a second's hesitation we urgently weaved our way through the maze of figures and flung our arms about each other. My fears were groundless. Our first separation had stood the test of time. We had a wonderful month together as a family again. Ted only had to say his usual greeting to Anthony: 'Anthony, where are you?' and Anthony clambered on to his knee and fell asleep being 'perked' (Ted twirling his fingers around Anthony's ears, which he had always adored and had been a night-time treat.) Ted burst into laughter when he first saw our rickety cottage, but he soon warmed to it.

Anthony was still awakening before dawn so, armed with buckets, spades and beachball, we headed off to nearby Joss Bay, unspoilt, extremely beautiful and backed by high cliffs. On the beach, washed clean by the sea, we raced with Anthony between us, leaving a six-footed trail, four large and two small, our shadows elongated by the rising sun. Ted and Anthony played ball and fearlessly Anthony chased it into the licking foam. On dull days out came the wellies and Anthony's fisherman pants. Intrepidly he would wade out into the spent waves or, hand-in-hand between us, clamber over the sharp rocks to peer at the pools left as the sea went back to France. We thought he would enjoy collecting shells, but not Anthony. He was more attracted to the varieties of seaweed, some brown, thick, slimy and pungent, others green and pregnant like distended peapods. Sea-blown, fresh and sand-dabbed, clutching our seaweed, we returned to the car and headed for home.

When Ted had to return to Australia I felt the ache of loneliness. I had soldiered on for Anthony's sake, but that first night alone, as I rolled into the pillow where Ted had been, I just wanted to be a woman again, warmed in the arms of the man she loved, in our carefree days before Anthony was born. Jolted from my dreams into reality the next morning, I curled with guilt at the fleeting moment the night before of wishing Anthony had never been born.

On fine mornings we still took Anthony to the beach, but his zest had waned as he looked vacantly out to sea or around him, expectantly, as if any moment his Daddy would appear. But Ted didn't and the time came when my little man refused to even get out of the car when we reached the beach. I tried to love him more, if that was possible, to compensate for our loss.

In the late summer of 1974, Christine Garbutt, of *Reveille* newspaper, wrote a feature about our struggle, our way of life and about the aims of our medical project. This article led me to meet the Watson family.

In August of that year, Angela Watson, their daughter, had a severe nosebleed after running in a race at her father's works' Sports Day. She was admitted to the Middlesex Hospital and doctors diagnosed severe aplastic anaemia. Placed in isolation, Brian and Sue Watson watched in anguish and despair at her rapid deterioration. The answer was a bone marrow transplant, but no members of Angela's family, not even her two brothers, matched. It appeared hopeless.

It was on one evening, returning from visiting Angela, that Brian read the article in *Reveille*. He asked Angela's doctor to contact Dr James. There was a chance that our donor register, even in its infancy, would have a donor for Angela. The computer, in fact, produced several. A perfect match was an 18-year-old local girl, Kathy Goodhew, one of the first registered in a donor session at Margate Hospital. The *Daily Express* ran a front-page feature on the transplant as a beautiful and brave teenager stepped forward unhesitatingly to try to save Angela. Bone marrow was taken from the donor, Kathy, under general anaesthetic, sucked out into a hollow needle from the chest or hip bones. This healthy marrow was dripped into Angela's bloodstream, hopefully to re-colonise in the bones and produce healthy blood cells.

While I was anxiously waiting to hear of Angela's progress, I was surprised to receive a visit from Mr Watson, his two young sons, his brother, Kathy (Angela's donor) and her father. We chatted in the car park at the side of the Jolly Farmer pub. As our second winter's isolation had begun (it was the beginning of November, 1974) I could not ask them into the cottage. Mr Watson had come personally to thank me for enabling Angela to have this chance to live.

I had seen the tragic photograph of Angela in the *Daily Express*, smiling bravely out of her sealed glass cubicle to her Mum and Dad. Her lovely face was thin and drawn, her eyes deeply shadowed and her hair limp and scant. One side effect of a bone marrow transplant is that the patient loses their hair. Fortunately this regrows when the crisis is over. Mr Watson produced a photo of Angela just a few months previously, a fitting name bestowed upon an angelic, beaming, beautiful girl, her round face rimmed by a halo of luxuriant light blonde hair. We talked quietly together. Mr Watson was worried they may have found Kathy too late. Angela had developed an abscess in the abdomen which was causing problems during her immuno-suppression. All we could do was hope and pray that it was not too late.

Of all the parents of sick children I have met I admire Mr and Mrs Watson and their families most of all. In this time of anguish for Angela they could still think of my son and other children in the future who needed the same help. They began fundraising in their area, Gravesend in Kent, and formed the first area branch of the Anthony Nolan Appeal. Each evening Mr Watson – I now called him Brian – would phone, or I would phone him to discuss Angela's condition. Kathy's donor cells rejected, so a second donor was quickly used, but Angela was extremely weak and beginning to show signs of grave stress, being locked in her cubicle for so long and unable to be in physical contact with her parents. They could kiss her only through the glass screen.

A few days later, one Saturday in November, Brian rang to tell me Angela was dead. The strain had been too much. Hysterical, she had screamed to be let out of her cubicle and had died of a heart attack. I hadn't really cried since leaving Australia. When tears threatened, I usually bit my bottom lip hard. Tears wouldn't solve anything had been my maxim. Anthony was asleep upstairs. I told Mum the tragic news. Slumped at the kitchen table, my head on my arms, I silently wept.

Only those who have truly grieved will understand when I say I didn't sob or scream, only wept, the tears welling over and over until I felt drained. I went to Angela's funeral bearing a wreath in the shape of the letter A, with the words 'From Anthony to Angela.' Kathy was far too upset from all she had been through to attend and was represented by her father. We gathered at Mr Watson's home, and I added my tribute to the hundreds of others, a display of such colour, perfume and splendour in memory of a child. I thought, what does one say on such an occasion? Words would not bring Angela back, but Angela had become a part of my adopted family of sick children. I was numbed with her loss. We had all tried so hard to save her. But Brian and Sue Watson were wonderful. They had their two little boys (both under nine) at school. It would all be over by the time they returned. They had a nickname for Angela, 'Missy'. Brian showed me photos and I was able in those few moments to watch a baby girl pass from a toddler to a lovely girl of six, now held in time's palm to be forever six. With such pride they showed me the beautiful photos of Angela laughing. The lounge was full of photographs and flowers. I thought to myself that I could not stand it if it had been Anthony. I couldn't. I couldn't look at a photograph of him ever again. I would have to keep his memory inside of me. But Brian helped me, displaying such calm and courage that day. He showed me Missy's room, untouched, her clothes and toys fruitlessly awaiting her return.

'What can you say, Shirley?' he said. 'I don't understand, do you?' I was too choked to reply, and just shook my head. 'She must have gone to Heaven,' he said. 'She was so lovely. I have two sons. Why couldn't God have taken one of my boys and not my little girl? But how could I choose which one? God only knows,' he sighed. And it must be so.

I followed in the first car behind Angela. I'd never attended a funeral before and this, my first, was the death of a child. The tiny coffin was hidden by the myriads of flowers. There were teddies and dolls made out of flowers, gazing lifelessly back at us through the windows. Such profound artistry and beauty for Angela, yet she could not see. We all tried so hard to control ourselves and painfully suppressed racking sobs and averted our faces and brushed away the tears. If we had been of another culture we could have mourned as one, called out our grief to the heavens. But each of us summoned control, thinking then that we would support each other. I thought back to the night I had howled like an animal in the shower in the maternity hospital at the thought of the death of my son.

It was cold at the funeral and the heavens grieved with us. A drizzly rain fell that grey November day as we entered the church. The ceremony was short and poignant. I listened to the words and squeezed my eyes to try to pray and stem the tears. But they opened, drawn again and again to the tiny coffin in the centre of the aisle. The parson spoke gently, the organ played and we sang the hymn, 'All Things Bright and Beautiful,' and I wanted to scream: No, damn it, no!

Approaching the cemetery a lank mourner, top hat and tailcoat glistening wet, stepped forward to guide the procession to the burial place. It was a page from Dickens; his thin, wet hair, his hunched, bony shoulders and hooked nose, stepping a familiar route. Angela's grave was beside her grandfather's. It was to be a triple grave, Brian told me, so that he and Sue would join Angela in the future. We gathered about the graveside as the drizzle abated and the last prayers were read ... ashes to ashes, dust to dust. I thought my head would explode.

I wept openly. As the coffin disappeared into the ground and flowers were strewn after it, Sue echoed my silent words and screamed aloud. 'No, God, no,' she cried. Brian firmly steered her away. I remember it all so vividly.

Brian and Sue, their family and friends still do tremendous work at our Gravesend branch to help reach a day when it may never happen again. And the Anthony Nolan Laboratories have a special room housing a very special microscope to aid our work in memory of Angela Watson.

Chapter 9

The media and the public mourned Angela and the subsequent publicity directed attention even more to Anthony's plight. I received more and more letters which kept me busy sometimes through the night until Anthony awoke in the early hours. I had to fit in more TV, radio and press interviews until I thought I would crack under the pressure. And the more I had to do for the Appeal, the more mother had to compensate by running the home and loving Anthony. I could still not leave him for more than a few hours, as he would allow only me to bathe, feed and administer his drugs. But he loved his Nanna best to nurse and sing to him. I always felt drained after an interview. I had to tell the same tragic story of Anthony over and over again.

When an event in our lives has caused grief or suffering, it is human nature to wish to forget. Dwelling on a tragedy eats like cancer and just as effectively destroys. We try to push it to the back of our minds, busy ourselves until time eases the pain of remembering. I have never been allowed to do this. The wound of my suffering has been opened so many times my memory is pulsing raw. The late nights dealing with Anthony's horrific haemorrhages and the psychological hammering or reliving over and over again his suffering left me pale and drawn. The only sleep I could manage was that induced by numerous sleeping pills. As I placed my head on my pillow, aching for sleep, the day's events flashed in a pageant behind my closed, flickering lids and my head burned with plans of all I had to achieve in the future. The sleeping pills planed the edges of my anxiety enough to slide me into oblivion, but I could, and had to, still wake instantly alert to cope with any emergency. I realised I couldn't cope for much longer at this pace. Each time I told the story I lived it. Now I erected an invisible barrier between the me before and the me now, so that when in interviews I related the events I wasn't talking about Shirley and Anthony Nolan, but fictitious characters in a drama. It could all be left behind by walking out the studio doors. This way it didn't seem to hurt so much. I could fix my mask for the cameras, modulate my voice for the recorders and peel and close them off at the end. I know that sometimes after particularly gruelling interviews, when an unintentionally piercing question such as, 'What will you do when Anthony dies?' had snap-frozen me for a split second, and Anthony's and Angela's funeral were as one, I almost burst into a sobbing and inarticulate heap. But instead, I raised my head, faced the people and said: 'He isn't going to die.' As a result, I have heard myself described as 'hard' but I am only as hard as a crustacean, its exterior essential to protect its interior, its life. Similarly, the constant fear of losing Anthony beat me as brutally as a storm-tossed boat against a cliff face. I felt torn to shreds and I believe, in the same way, I also erected a barrier between me and Anthony to enable me to deal with his illness and try to find a donor to save him.

A nurse or a doctor can't take on the suffering of each patient. They have to close themselves off to a degree to be of positive help. I had to think positively, not negatively. Yes, I hardened. I had to if we were to survive – and Anthony has survived so far.

As the days rolled by in the monotony of our isolation, towards Anthony's third birthday, each day in winter appeared the same. The early hours of play, the walks and the apparently endless hours cramped in a tiny cottage. We could have no close human contact because of the influenza threat which could prove fatal to Anthony. We could briefly, while out on our walks, talk to villagers or passers-by, but no one could enter the cottage. Nor could we visit anyone. Peter delivered our food from next door. Anthony's entire world was mother, myself and his tiny home. An interview now became a welcome event, a change from the routine. I could also enjoy the off-camera conversation and share a joke with the crews. They were wonderful to Anthony, bringing him gifts which they knew I could wash or disinfect. Anthony loved the pretty lights and flashes and was fascinated by the mechanics, the booms, clapper boards, recording equipment and the cameras most of all. We re-entered our cottage and waved them off, leaving them blue-faced, red-nosed, shoulder-thumping and finger-blowing, but reflecting Anthony's smile after their winter's hike. For the first time in winter I allowed a cameraman and photographer to enter the cottage to record the miracle of Anthony's third birthday. They were prepared in the yard by donning gowns, masks and shoe covers. The familiar cameras calmed an instant reaction by Anthony at the sight of the hospital masks and, seated at his own little table, his birthday cake in the shape of a figure 3 before him, we lit his candles and he blew them out and cheered with glee. 'Again, again,' he called as the three melted candles were replaced and his joyful hip-hip-hoorays shook the walls to the accompaniment of the two cameramen, happily sweating under lights and behind lenses.

Anthony's third birthday pictures appeared in newspapers all over the world and on national television. It was a salute, his triumph so far over all prognosis. Of course, Anthony would not be eating any part of his beautiful cake. I wrapped it carefully and stored it, deciding to keep it as a talisman to be taken out at his fourth birthday. I was to do exactly that, unknowingly setting a pattern for other birthdays in isolation when the old cake would appear to join the new number and both be alight again with hope and faith. At the end of the day I would destroy the old cake and store the new.

* * *

I noticed for the first time on the birthday photographs how pale and drawn mother looked. Being in such close contact for so long, my attention mainly directed towards Anthony, I had failed to realise how ill she was. She had mentioned that her back ached, but I had assumed it was the chill, damp weather. Soon she was gritting her teeth, racked with pain as she moved. She refused to sit down and continued her usual routine chores, only now she couldn't lift Anthony and he couldn't understand why. That evening, I made her a hot drink and gave her analgesics. She brushed aside my suggestion to call her doctor and slowly, painfully, climbed the stairs, pulling herself up by the banister, aided and supported behind by me.

The next morning I found her rigid with pain. She could not even hold the cup of tea I had brought for her. I called her doctor who came some hours later. Gazing abruptly and haughtily about our humble cottage, he stated she had a slipped disc and should lie as still as possible. He scribbled on his prescription pad and, over his shoulder, descending the steep stairs, said, 'If she is no better in a week get her to lie on the floor on the boards.' I stood holding the scrap of paper in my hand. How could I even get her prescription? I couldn't leave Anthony. Behind me mother was quietly weeping. For mother to cry for herself she must be ill, I thought. Anthony kept toddling up the stairs and trying to drag his Nanna out of bed. He couldn't understand why she wasn't up and about as usual.

I had to prop mother on pillows for her to even manage to sip a hot drink and, at the same time, keep a watchful eye on Anthony's every move. Now an active toddler, the stairs were a hazardous attraction. Mother couldn't leave her bed to wash or go to the toilet. Just to touch her made her wince, as if every nerve-ending was raw. After 48 hours I was worried, exhausted and afraid. I knew she needed to be in hospital. Yet how would Anthony react? His Nanny had barely left him in three years. How would I manage alone? I knew that a slipped disc could take weeks to resettle by the old method of lying on boards, and, during that time, the patient suffers immense pain and discomfort. I also knew that Anthony was unwittingly causing mother more pain by trying to pull her out of bed. I phoned mother's doctor and, speaking the password 'private patient,' arranged that evening for her to see a specialist.

She was admitted to hospital immediately and put on traction. Her pain was eased with a quick injection. Eight days later she was able to return home. She was not allowed to lift at all and wore a supporting belt for her back but she could walk and nurse Anthony on her lap. She was on the mend.

The eight days without her had been hell. Anthony pined for his Nanna and I barely managed to cope single-handed. We were both shadows of our former selves, but I had learned one lesson – there's one rule for the rich and one for the poor. Somehow we scraped and paid the doctor's bills. While mother was in hospital I had written to Ted in Australia of our struggle. I didn't know how long mother would be ill and I expressed my belief that it was impossible for me to nurse and care for Anthony, run the Appeal and keep the cottage, simulating reverse barrier nursing procedure indefinitely. He decided to sell our home in Australia and return to England.

During this period under pressure I received encouraging news that the government's working party had presented their report to the Minister and recommended the funding of research and development in the field of bone marrow transplant. I was elated and optimistic that now my tremendous responsibility of funding our medical project would be alleviated. I was finding it increasingly difficult to carry on alone with the Appeal.

However, the recommendation never came to fruition. In the spring of 1975 the transplant team was informed that due to Britain's economic recession no money was available. Cutbacks were recommended and implemented by the National Health Service. Wards were closed, geriatric units closed, staff pruned. As the axe fell, waiting lists for operations and treatments grew longer and longer. It was a disgusting soul-destroying policy, yet British Leyland, due to strikes, could be bailed out of insolvency at a cost of many millions. None of it made any sense to me. The public, bless 'em, continued their wonderful support and enabled our donor testing programme to continue.

Just before Christmas, 1974, my attention had been drawn once again to the political scene by the arrival in Britain of Australia's Prime Minister, Gough Whitlam. Extremely bitter because of the bureaucratic flack shot by two governments whenever they were approached for answers by the people, and because they always had the skill to parry the lances of truth, I decided to try to meet our leaders personally. Through friends, I knew Mr Whitlam's itinerary. I prepared placards with photographs of Anthony bloodsmeared during a haemorrhage. These photographs had been taken the day after his third birthday with an ordinary instamatic camera, still loaded partly with shots of the joyous birthday cheers. The placards were headed 'The British and Australian Governments are letting Anthony Nolan die.'

Helped by a handful of students from Ramsgate, we quietly prepared to enter Downing Street. Our way was barred by policemen. We barely had time to hold those placards of a bloodied Anthony towards the fleet of expensive cars bearing Gough Whitlam and his entourage, turning into Downing Street, before I was abruptly confronted by a tight-lipped, immaculately dressed official from No. 10. I was questioned, guarded on either side by police. What was my name? My age? My religion? Where was I born? Which school did I attend? and so it went on. We had not uttered a word. We had not shouted or waved our placards. We had simply been there; a silent condemnation, to try to bring to the attention of our leaders, so-called representatives of the people, the plight of one small boy ... to try to obtain for him all they promised in their pre-electoral political party parcels. Where was Anthony's right even to live in our society?

I was escorted to Scotland Yard and the questions continued. I was registered as a demonstrator for holding up my dying child to our governments.

The London bobbies were wonderful, gentle and courteous. One on either side. They said they had followed Anthony's struggle and they wished me well. As the questions were completed, I was allowed to leave, and, tongue-in-cheek, my interrogator said: 'Oh, by the way, madam, if you wish to lodge a complaint, it's Chief Inspector Greene with an "e".'

Some years later the entire metropolitan police force were to step forward as volunteer donors to try to save Anthony. I met up again with my placard-bearers in a cafe next to Westminster Underground Station, and over a quick lunch planned my next move. I wasn't giving in at one attempt. Leaving the lads, I hailed a cab to the Park Lane Hotel. I brushed past the doorman and at the reception desk calmly asked to see Prime Minister Whitlam. A call from his suite asked me to wait in the foyer. As the wealthy paraded before me I waited patiently, to no avail. I had entered into conversation with an eccentric and devastatingly wealthy elderly American lady who was about to leave for Heathrow to fly back to the United States in her husband's company plane. We had spent a stimulating and amusing hour together when she said, 'Are you waiting for someone, my dear?' 'Yes,' I replied with aplomb, 'the Australian Prime Minister!'

I approached the reception desk again and again and eventually two burly chaps appeared through the lift doors. They questioned me, discreetly, not wishing to draw attention in the domain of the affluent. Just as discreetly I expressed my desire to speak with the Prime Minister. I was told he was resting and unavailable. These were his personal bodyguards and they were extremely puzzled how I knew Mr Whitlam's arrival time at Downing Street and at which hotel he was staying. I declined to enlighten them. They turned on their heels and disappeared as abruptly as they had appeared. So much for Mr Whitlam the humanitarian ...

My last attempt was the Prime Minister's arrival at Australia House. Silent but determined, we stood beside the placards. The police made no attempt to move us on and many passers-by stopped to read the placards and leaflets, look at the photographs and offer words of encouragement. But just as quietly and effectively, obviously planned during the afternoon, the police formed a human screen as the Prime Minister entered and left the building. I doubt if he even knew of our presence. I often wonder now if he would even care. From Britain he was going on to France for a meeting with French officials to try to dissuade them from further testing of nuclear weapons in the Pacific. I was particularly interested in this part of his European visit, as one theory put forward for Anthony's rare blood disorder was that it could have been caused by a genetic mutation due to radiation. Mr Whitlam was totally unsuccessful. Many more tests followed and their side effects were politically and effectively played down.

As night closed in and the bright city lights blinked and illuminated Aldwych, our breath fogged our faces. Cold and tired after our demonstration we headed back to Kent. Soon afterwards, Prime Minister Whitlam was speeding back to Australia due to destruction of Darwin by Cyclone Tracey. We had lived in Darwin and feared for the safety of many dear friends. We were preparing for our second Christmas alone in England when we heard the news of the tragedy. I was aghast at the TV shots of the devastated city. Ted knew just what I would be thinking and telephoned to reassure me that our friends were unharmed.

He also told me that our Adelaide house had been sold and he expected to be with us by the end of January. Despite mother's frailty, my fruitless attempts in London, and the shock of Darwin's destruction, as the hours closed on 1974 we looked with more optimism to 1975, cheered by the lusty strains of Auld Lang Syne from the Jolly Farmer pub. As the clock pointed to midnight we raised our glasses to toast the New Year and smiled those first seconds into 1975.

I thought: Please God, this year may we find Anthony's donor and may he be cured.

* * *

We had now lived in the cottage just over a year; winter had started early and once again the persistent rain meant that for most of the time we were indoors. The two downstairs rooms measured approximately 12 feet by 10 feet and the stairs cut through the middle. There was not even enough space to fix a door so they rose steeply up to mother's bedroom on the left and the bathroom on the right. I had had an inside loo fitted in preparation for this second winter. The first winter's expeditions across the back yard in rain, snow and slop had made this a top-priority job. Another smaller flight of stairs led to Anthony's bedroom at the front of the cottage and mine at the rear. It was, in fact, an ideal cottage for a retired couple. We had worked hard making it attractive and cosy. But it was not suited to a toddler.

As soon as my back was turned Anthony was up the stairs like a lizard up a tree. I had a safety gate, but only fixed it at night at the top of the stairs in case Anthony climbed out of his cot. To fix it during the day was to place bars inside a prison. While Mum did all the chores I gave Anthony my undivided attention and the cottage was his unquestionable domain. I had decided that now our home in Australia was sold I must look for a bigger cottage with a large garden where Anthony could safely play. He was becoming more and more adventurous, no longer content to toddle down the quiet country lanes. He wanted to explore the larger main road, a hazardous recreation due to the continuous flow of heavy transports hauling cars to and fro from Ramsgate Harbour.

While Ted was selling our belongings and packing up in Australia I again contacted estate agents and began the search for a better home for Anthony. I was looking for a property similar to our present cottage, only with more interior space and a garden. It would also have to be inexpensive, which would mean, as we knew only too well, hard work again renovating. After paying off our mortgages in Australia there would not be a great deal left over. I awaited each morning the plop of the agent's envelope on the mat and eagerly opened and scanned the contents. Most were too expensive and any which appeared potentially suitable sent me careering off in the little old Ford to be first at the agent's office.

This is how I discovered Leeside at Challock Lees, in the beautiful weald of Kent. It was a sprawling, tumbling timber cottage, stone-dash covered. Sitting aged and alone between the woods at the rear and the village green or Lees at the front, it had, I later discovered been a World War One army hut. Any normal house buyer would not have ventured through the front gate hanging on its rusty hinges, displaying the barely visible nameplate, Leeside.

In the sharp January morning, cracking and spattering iced puddles, I bumped along the unmade track parallel to the road to Canterbury leading to the cottage and clambered out. I noted the village green, the neighbouring houses – large, expensive, pseudo-Georgian, but a good distance from the cottage. I rubbed away at the dirty windows and peered into the darkened rooms. Yes, I noted the rotted sills and the plaster fallen away in places revealing the original timber structure, but as I paced it out the cottage length was 63 feet long (the original hut structure) by 15 feet wide. At some later stage an additional room had been added, making it an L-shape.

Struggling through a tangle of ivy and broken glass I found that a verandah and conservatory graced the east side. I could see in my mind's eye just what we could do with this forsaken cottage. As I brushed the dirt and frost from my nose and the cobwebs from my shoulders I thought, well, you've mastered concreting, painting and decorating once, now here's a real challenge!

Trekking through the knee-length grass round the garden sealed the bond. Even in its decay, its wilderness, it was appealing. The rear garden was large and flat and I could already see Anthony next summer, running free about the apple trees. The view to the south was breathtaking. Rows of young nursery trees, bare, supple hands reaching to spring; and beyond, shades of green, beautiful conifers, as far as the eye could see. In my eagerness to drive into Ashford to the estate agent, I reversed my car on to the village green, deceived by the first frost, and believing the land hard. I was soon disillusioned. The mud sucked greedily at the tyres, spinning ineffectively. Lesson number one learned in rural Challock; I slipped and slopped across the Lees to the garage opposite. It needed a Land Rover to tow me out.

Ted came home to us the next day. Stopping off on our way from Heathrow to Manston, I showed him Leeside; he approved of the cottage. Weeks of renovation lay ahead, but this was to be our new home. Having Ted home again generated conflicting reactions. It was reassuring to have him beside me, yet in those first few days we were like strangers. We had been apart now for one-and-a-half years, and during that time he had been leading a normal life. Mum and I, in contrast, had been striving to keep Anthony alive. We were almost fanatical in our attempts to avoid infection. I recall I even phoned the estate agent from the garage to ask if the keys were available for viewing, and at the same time asked if he had a cold.

Ted wasn't used to living this totally restricted and selfless life. I believe he didn't fully understand the sacrifice it would involve to be with us again. It's impossible to relate to an experience and all it entails simply by reading about it. To be fully aware of how we felt, how and why we behaved as we did, he would need to have been with us. Ted was tanned from the Australian summer, vibrant and healthy; we were pale and tired, our nerves raw. He wanted to go across to the pub and take me out to dinner and drive up to London to visit his family and old friends. I would have loved to step out of those winter confines, but I had a loyalty to Anthony. In the middle of the influenza season I was not going to let the temptation of my pleasure be responsible for killing my only child. I knew that I also had a loyalty to Ted but what choice did I have? Anthony was defenceless and desperately ill.

Each day we literally walked a knife-edge between life and death. I had to put Anthony first. Ted was like having a friendly lion underfoot, pacing the tiny cottage; he simply didn't understand. How could he? He had been away a long time and he expected to be fussed over. Yet the preparing of meals, the extra washing, the physical demands as a wife, were just too much. I barely managed to get through an average day with Anthony and the Appeal, let alone make room in it for a demanding third.

As soon as Anthony was in bed, I began answering letters in the quiet of the kitchen. Mother went straight to bed. I remember an amusing quip of hers one evening on retiring. 'If Prince Charming and a coach-and-four were to pull up at this cottage to take me out I would decline and go to bed,' she said. Our greatest desire was sleep. I averaged about six hours usually, and I used to be a 10-hour or grouchy type. Ted would switch on the TV and settle, naturally, to relax for an evening's normal entertainment.

This was not a normal house; it was Anthony's world. I found the babble distracting, being already tired before I began the paperwork, and mother was disturbed in her bedroom immediately above. With the thin boards she may just as well have been resting her head on the TV. This is not a condemnation ... this is how Anthony's illness had affected us. We were geared like detonators to trigger at any sound, and the TV with its reflection of the outside world – the fun, the laughter, its fantasia – all appeared a mockery of our existence.

The purchase of the cottage at Challock was completed and we began work. Mother and I went alternate days with Ted to work on it; we preferred the day's renovating to remaining behind as the physical labour was a release. Our willingness to go to a day's navvying – be it demolishing, digging, concreting or decorating in below-zero temperatures – obviously reflected our repressed desire to be released from the confines of isolation. A new home to look forward to, the change of routine, and the fresh air and exercise brought our psychological and physical improvement. The cottage was being completely geared for Anthony. Steps were removed and those too steep were made into slopes. We were trying to create a larger and more interesting world in which he could be released and develop and play in safety. Some interior doors were removed to create larger play areas. I thought the long hallway, originally a corridor in the army hut, would be smashing for a game of football during bad weather. We knocked out a small latch window and put in French windows opening directly on to the garden to encourage

Anthony, hopefully, out to play. Mother built a large sandpit in the base of an old shed we had demolished, barrowing piles of left-over sand. It was all for Anthony.

Yet, on reflection, those weeks he was left with one or other of us must have inflicted further irreparable psychological damage. In winter Anthony had the close human contact of only two people, mother and I. A child able to lead a normal life has the contact of numerous close friends and sometimes hundreds of others, such as periodic visits by relatives or friends, and the chance to explore shops, supermarkets, villages, towns; ride buses, trains, merry-go-rounds; to go to school, the cinema, a pantomime or funfair. Yet Anthony could do none of these. Being away for several weeks preparing the cottage we were taking away each day half of his world. Despite our love and our efforts to stimulate him, the monotony of his walks along now-empty wintry lanes and the long hours in the cottage in poor weather caused further regression. It was little more than an isolation cubicle multiplied by six.

We worked on frantically as Anthony's behaviour became more erratic. His tantrums would cause Ted to attempt to discipline him and this in turn acted as a catalyst for argument. My immediate reaction was always to protect Anthony; he was so frail he bruised at the slightest knock. The tantrums were a cry for help, a demand for attention in his empty life. Anthony was too young to comprehend an explanation of why we left him for so long each day, when we had never left him before. I was wrong to argue in front of Anthony, which only added to his distress and confusion. Perhaps once again he saw his abandonment, Ted's animosity and my agitation as further punishment.

I had hoped having his daddy back with us would be of help to Anthony, especially regarding his disinterest in food. At three-and-a-half-years he was still wearing the same size clothes and shoes he had worn in Australia two years previously. He was still bathed in the same baby bath before the fire as if his tiny flickering life was suspended, a child forever, yet ironically deprived of most of the joys of childhood; locked away from the world as time marched on and left him behind.

Somehow Ted failed him. Anthony reached out but somehow Ted seemed unable to give what was needed. Ted, I knew, thought we were too lenient with Anthony and saw his role as the new disciplinarian. But what 'harder punishment can be inflicted on a child than imprisonment? If a normal child misbehaves it is sent to its room for a limited period. The punishment is the deprivation of freedom. Most of Anthony's life he had been denied the freedom to be a child, to walk free with other children, and I desperately wanted to keep him alive to do just that. At the same time I was battling government ignorance and apathy and also funding Dr James' medical project. I was doing what I thought was best; there was no one to guide me ... no other child with Anthony's condition had ever survived this long.

Years later, back in Australia, the words of our child and family psychiatrist captured the episode: 'It's people that count, not places. It's who you're with, not where you are.' We could have possibly helped Anthony more those winter months by being with him, not preparing a larger cage.

Waiting. I was always waiting for a directive from Westminster Hospital that a compatible donor had been found at last. Hoping Anthony would have his transplant while the Challock cottage was being prepared for him and when he was cured come home to our love, freedom and spring. This is how I kept going day to day, hoping and praying Anthony's donor would soon be found.

By Easter we hacked our way through several feet of snow up the driveway to the cottage. The work had to go on but through frosted leaf windowpanes, warm-breath washed, it was hard not to stop the sanding or painting to peer out at the Christmas card scene of giant firs, their bent boughs blooming with mock blossoms, at hedges, ice-cream topped and grass blade tips snow-brushed, curled as delicate as the snowdrops they preceded.

With white frosted breath I crunched my track to the giant apple tree and scattered the remains of my sandwich pack on to the bird table, placed there by a previous unknown dweller. All was white, pure and silent. The rounded mounds, nature's muffler, had softened the edges of winter. I raised my face to the snow clouds bursting, pregnant-heavy, to the myriads of snowflakes mutated to black specks by my vertical gaze and felt them brush and melt like tears on my cheeks and eyelashes. I closed my eyes, drank the icy fresh air and knew a moment of peace.

The interior was completed by early May but we could proceed no further. Our money was gone. Everything had cost more than we had anticipated. We were too proud to apply for social security and the jobs available for Ted, used to running his own small business, were poorly paid in comparison with past earnings in Australia. He decided to return to Australia as he felt he could support us better from there.

The exterior as yet was untouched, the garden a wilderness. But the cottage was habitable. The rest could wait. We had fitted flat acrylic carpet, in blended tones of brown, which could be scrubbed and wouldn't show the stains of Anthony's haemorrhages. The panelled walls were a soothing beige and the beams and frames were black. The whole effect was homely and 'olde worlde'.

The only furniture we had bought was a three-piece suite, a Chesterfield, rounded and soft for Anthony's protection. We were pleased with our labours. The cottage had charm, character and space, lots and lots of space, all on one level for Anthony. But would he like it? Would he accept it? How would he react, yet again, to a strange new world?

Ted had to leave in a few days and I didn't want his departure to coincide with our move. We were now familiar with every nook and cranny of the cottage but Anthony had yet to be introduced to it. We hired a van and moved our beds and few bits of furniture from Manston while Anthony had his daily nap. Over the months we had the open fires ablaze, one in the lounge and one in the dining room, and also had a powerful mobile gas heater which we moved from room to room as we worked. Coal had been ordered for the open fires and the old stove in the kitchen, which heated the water and several antiquated, but effective, radiators. Leaving the coal fires glowing and the stove muttering and grumbling at being raked out of retirement, we returned to Manston to collect Anthony, his cot and Mum. Once again in the same old Ford, its roof rack a collage of an emptied home, we headed for Leeside.

Ted drove while I nursed Anthony, whose face was a mixed expression of resignation and expectation. Mum sat in the back seat beside the kettle, teapot and cups, always her first and last consideration on any move. We turned into the driveway, still thinly snow-covered. At barely four p.m. the clear cool evening was drawing in. I bustled Anthony into the cottage and, heart in my mouth, exhausted from lifting beds and boxes, geared myself to find a reserve of energy and patience to deal with his expected distress. The cottage was warm and welcoming as the lights flickered on. Anthony blinked like a tiny barn owl, stared about him, hesitated and, face abeam, toddled up and down the lengthy hallway. I felt immense relief as he eagerly began exploring each room. Ted and Mum unloaded the car and, while Ted assembled Anthony's cot, mother busied herself making a pot of tea. I allowed myself to fold on to the comfy settee before the blazing fire and stretched my feet to toast by the fender.

Book Two

Chapter 10

As spring quickly severed the bonds of winter, so Ted abruptly left one warm day at the end of May. I felt a severing of our bond, an ending of that special something we had shared before Anthony had been born. Children do change a relationship and the effect is usually polarised. There are those couples who bloom a second time in the shared love and joy of their offspring and those who resent their intrusion. Children are not all powder-soft, clean, and gurgling happily as they are in TV commercials. They can, and do, stretch nerves raw when they are teething and a good night's sleep becomes a thing of the past. They enjoy being noisy, dirty and sometimes so strong-willed you could throttle them. I had become a mother; Ted had never become a father. He had missed Anthony's development from babyhood to being a toddler. Unwittingly, Anthony was an irritant and a rival for my attention. I was disappointed that Ted didn't seem inclined to make up for lost time by romping and playing with Anthony. To him, being a father was being a provider in the material sense; a roof over our head and food in our stomach, but something indefinable was missing. I confess that it was with relief that I waved goodbye as he disappeared into the departure lounge at Heathrow. With an increased sense of purpose I headed the car for home.

At the same time as this period of moving into a larger cottage I was working closely with Marian Matthews. Marian had written a good deal of first-rate material during Simon's transplant and was keenly interested in this medical breakthrough. She had followed Simon's progress and, just as keenly, ours. From Anthony's third birthday photographs she obtained the negative of a good shot from Nick Skinner, with whom she worked. During long telephone conversations we planned a leaflet and letterhead paper for the Appeal. A block for printing was made of this photograph, depicting Anthony, chubby and beautiful, cheering over his birthday cake. Marian arranged the printing at cost at the nearby Chesham Press in Buckinghamshire, who have supported us from our inception. Leaflets and letterheads saved a tremendous amount of time writing explanatory letters. Unpaid, Marian shared with me the mammoth task of answering the thousands of letters. As the leaflets were gradually sent out that spring of 1975 we were sowing seeds of enlightenment, many of which fell on fruitful ground and generated tremendous interest and support.

The laboratory technicians had now tested and registered over 5,000 bone marrow donors and Dr James was invited to lecture in many parts of the world, including Sydney, Australia, at the Ninth Annual Congress of World Pathologists, where he presented his paper on our project entitled 'The First 5,000.' He then went on to Auckland, New Zealand, which proved propitious later, in several ways. I thought that first 5,000 a very long way from 50,000 but it *was* the first rung on the ladder and I now had several loyal individuals and groups working with me.

The many letters arriving at Westminster Hospital soon became too much for Marian and me and it became essential to employ a laboratory secretary, Mrs Betty Tobey. Betty recorded the thousands of volunteer donors on completed donor forms stored in large files labelled in districts. The end of a passage with a desk across served as her office. It was soon bursting with large black files and Kent, London, Essex, Yorkshire, Ireland, Wales and other places stared back at me each time we liaised on Appeal business. Thousands of willing donors were waiting to be tested yet we were still limited by lack of facilities, space, limited funds, the number of technicians we could employ and, consequently, the number of volunteers we could test. Never a visit to Dr James or Betty passed when I did not stare at those files with the thought that one of them held Anthony's donor.

We were all hoping that Anthony would be lucky like Simon and find a donor speedily. We were a dedicated team working towards the day when a donor register existed so that a child's life didn't depend on luck and if a patient needed a donor it would be immediately available. I never wanted to witness again a child subjected to the lonely life of my little boy.

It was only a few months later I discovered there was one other little boy, David, 'the boy in a bubble' in America.

The heat of summer burst forth like the opening of a kiln door. Britain had not experienced such glorious weather in decades. Each morning, round as an orange and just as promising, the sun topped the giant conifers, a single giant fruit. Now we had a larger home my young cousin Linda was able to come to spend the summer with us and bring a little of the zest of the outside world to Anthony, something mother and I had lost in our serious and lonely struggle, and to be with mother to help care for Anthony when I attended to the increasing demands of the Appeal. We were out barefooted, making sand pies in Anthony's sandpit as early as seven a.m. or snaking trails in the cool grass, silvered by the morning dew. Round and round the huge old apple trees we went until we toppled, laughing, warm and damp-dappled beneath the boughs. As temperatures soared into the 90s we exulted in the light and warmth. Out came Anthony's inflatable pool on the patio and we cheered, chairing him in and out, swinging him high into the air then dipping him into the cool water. 'Again, do it again, Lindama,' he cried, mixing our two names. He had come to love Linda dearly. She was the only other person in his world, so far, with whom he had established close contact. He would drag her gently to her knees, placing his arms about her, ruffling her short curls. With his head placed on hers he would say, 'Ah! Linda, my Linda.'

In the afternoons we cavorted like foals. It was so hot we dressed only in light beach wear and Anthony was as naked as the day he was born. We used the garden hose on each other and this was Anthony's favourite game. As I thinned the force with my thumb to a sprinkle, he would run again and again under the spray, undeterred by the shock of cold water on hot flesh. We sizzled and baked bun-brown against the Mediterranean blue skies, and we were happy.

I always left my paperwork until night so that Anthony had my attention during his waking hours. Linda and mother would then amble at the end of the day across the village green to the lovely old Chequers Inn and sit outside and relax in those rich summer evenings to the scent of roses and the buzz of gnats. In the seclusion and charm of our old beamed dining room, serving also as my office and bedroom, I worked away, now deeply involved in something more than a struggle for my son's life, but for all he represented; the right of each individual for a chance to live, especially the rights of sick and deprived children who had little power to survive without our support.

Anthony's favourite flower is the daisy. Scattered about the lawn were clusters like confetti and he devised a game of chasing daisies, a sort of daisy garden hopscotch. We would run from one daisy patch to another, circling them, jumping over them with Anthony yelling, 'Some more daisies, some more and some more and some more,' as we chased about the lawn. When I mowed the grass with a power mower I developed muscles I didn't know I possessed, having to steer the heavy machine to avoid guillotining the daisies. A strange sight to visitors, our lawn, with tufts of grass like broom heads protecting Anthony's daisies.

As each hot day melted molten to a fiery sunset I picked up my tired toddler, warm and happily weary, and nursed him like a baby, his face flushed beneath the apple blossom, and sang again and again at his request, 'I'U give you a daisy a day, dear.' He was happy, tanned, active and interested, but still he didn't grow. Nor did his appetite improve. Yet his skin had improved beyond belief. I no longer had to bathe him in Condy's crystals nor plaster him with a variety of creams for eczema. It was now clear and soft, the only remnants being slightly swollen finger and toe joints. His hair was thick and shiny. Indeed, one problem was the battle of frequently needed haircuts to keep it under control. Not a tear in his eye, his screams for help would have merited any film Oscar! Trimmed, dressed and smelling that special fresh of a bathed toddler, I cuddled him, and told him his favourite story of The Three Bears until his eyelids drooped, and clutching 'Woof' he fell asleep.

While we played with Anthony in the sun one of us would work on the cottage or the garden. We gradually demolished large, rotten wooden garden sheds, or original ablution huts, by using them for fuel. Mother loved gardening and transformed the wilderness. A rubbish heap cleared became a rose garden and an uninteresting patio surround became landscaped curves of snowdrops, crocuses, daffodils, geraniums and irises as the seasons changed. Untidy hedgerows became neat backdrops for her flower borders. I restored the lawns and kept them cut, but the beauty of the garden was mother's creation.

Linda and I preferred paint brushes, and while Linda dabbed at the yards and yards of pebbledash, I painstakingly painted the many tiny window frames. The rotten square hut windows had been replaced by pseudo-Georgian bows that required patience and expertise to produce a neat finish. We worked happily in the sunshine.

Once Anthony had adjusted to his new home and had the added love of Linda, I was able to take part each week in some fundraising event. The wonderful Watson family always had some idea to raise money for the Appeal. I joined one of their sponsored walks in laps around the park and esplanade at Gravesend in Kent. It was a clear, hot day, the rolling bitumen paths shimmering in the heat-haze. I have to admit I completed only 10 miles of the 15-mile course; I must have been in worse physical condition that I thought, or my feet were.

I especially enjoyed the invitations to talk to schools. Feeling the invisible vibrations of the healthy energetic young about me, immediately I shed years and was once again the young, carefree schoolma'am striding happily to meet each new day. Many schools gave mammoth support, such as the London Boys' School at Blackfriars, the Lady Margaret School for Girls and the Northcliffe School for Girls. I could fill pages to thank these wonderful youngsters. They demonstrated that the majority of youth are caring, responsible individuals and not inarticulate pot-smoking bludgers.

I talked to ladies' groups in villages, towns and cities, to factories and licensees, and was given a warm reception everywhere. Many pubs and clubs up and down the country supported our Appeal, organising collections, raffles and sponsored darts matches. The larger clubs and hotels held concerts. The social clubs in the north of England are huge establishments and draw top world entertainers; they also drew entertainers and members in support of Anthony's struggle. So many groups and individuals stepped forward with love to help. In Belfast, Northern Ireland, in the midst of its death and destruction, a bunch of youngsters called Robins alone raised £2,000. A little girl of nine years raised £400 by a sponsored swim 70 lengths of an Olympic pool. Old-age pensioners sent their extra pence earned gardening; the coast guards, ambulance men, social dubs from all levels organised dances, barbeques, dinners, cheese and wine parties, football, rugby and cricket matches and marathon sponsored walks, one by a Castleford man in Yorkshire and another by two Leeds men who walked almost the length of England.

I always wrote to express my sincere and heartfelt thanks to all these wonderful people, and at last in these pages I can extend the same thanks to all those who actively supported our work and still do and have remained anonymous.

That year of 1975, I would stop for a fleeting moment during the day or night, awed and humbled, warmed by the knowledge that at that exact moment someone, somewhere was actively working to try to save my little boy. I have heard bitter criticism levelled at the media but to my son and me and our struggle, they were kind, courteous and concerned, and went to any lengths to be as helpful as possible. Without them and the interest they generated, I could have achieved nothing. I was able, with the good weather, to grant numerous requests for interviews worldwide; it was hard work, but Anthony still enjoyed the camera and the film crews. He would even jump eagerly asking for a flash again or direct the chaps to switch on their lights. In a way this was Anthony's funfair, a jolly bustling crowd, with laughter, lights and fun. He disliked the telephone and some press interviews ... my earnest discussion, my relating of past unhappy events, and my anger at faceless administrators was easily transmitted to my toddler who was now quickly learning to understand adult language. My demeanour alone was sufficient to relay my agitation, and almost protectively Anthony would try to pull me away from the telephone or the journalist.

As day followed after glorious day we were able to have more visitors. My younger brother Tony came during university vacation; my mother's sister, Doris, called frequently. Anthony eagerly looked forward to visits from his Auntie Dot D-Dot Dot; it was a long trek for her from industrial Yorkshire, but she loved to see her little lad. Roger de Courcy came, too, bringing his Nookey bear (as famous in Britain as Humphrey in Australia) to present a cheque for the Appeal after his participation in one of Neville Nisse's concerts.

One special visit I shall always remember: the second visit of Anthony's great-great-grandmother. She hadn't seen him for almost two years since his arrival. In her eighties, frail and determined, my Uncle Bob drove her down from Yorkshire with her mother's other sister, Anthony's Aunt Lily. We took photographs in the sun on the patio ... Anthony's family complete, except for his father and my dead grandfather. Anthony was ecstatic, chatting to them and dancing for them. He had people round him, people who loved him.

Adults were no infection risk when free from colds and influenza, but children and pets were, so Anthony's world was peopled with adults.

The only one noticeable effect was that Anthony bypassed a stage of oral development. From the Mumma, Dadda stage in Australia he didn't attempt to talk much from 1973 to 1975; when he did it wasn't the enchanting babble of baby talk, but adult phrases, adult words.

Sadly, he had once again missed being a child. He perhaps thought he was an adult and, in consequence, this generated immense frustration at being unable to compete in an all-adult world. I knew one day he would reach a stage when he stopped even trying; I was desperately racing to beat that time.

As a teacher, I realised the seriousness of his deprivation and made a point of playing at his levels, speaking with him, kneeling down and cutting the world down to his size. I would lift him up to show him the world beyond his reach ... mantelshelves, bookshelves, the cooker with the interesting bubbling, steaming pans, cooking food I knew he wouldn't eat. He examined the sink, loo, washing machine and fridge ... under my guidance I allowed him to explore all within a degree of safety. I taught him how to handle fire ... he had already mastered boxes of matches way back in the Manston cottage, learned to hold a box, strike a match, light a candle, blow out the match, and when it was cool he would say, 'It's dead, mummy,' and put it in the bin.

The open fires, solid fuel stove and gas fire made it essential that Anthony should realise their potential danger. He did and he never came to harm. If a cinder fell from the fire, even within the safety of the fireguard, he would call out to me.

With Anthony's haemorrhaging problem and lack of resistance to infection it was essential to avoid even the most minor accident. Today, in a moment of my forgetfulness, he will jolt me with, 'Mummy, Mummy, the kettle's boiling.'

* * *

The phone jangled, and the call brought hope. As I replaced the receiver I yelled, 'Mum, we may have a donor! I have to organise some blood samples for testing.'

My GP and his partner were in the next village, picturesque Wye. They were wonderful fellows, gentle, kind and helpful. Besides running a large and busy rural practice – they also manned a service with a specially equipped vehicle to dash to emergencies in farms, villages and accidents on the two large motorways that cut parallel scars across their territory.

That day the sequence began at eight a.m. All prepared with soap, towels and foot covers, we awaited their arrival. It took two doctors, a nurse and myself to hold Anthony, to bleed him successfully and to obtain sufficient test tubes of blood for donor compatibility tests. I always helped by talking to Anthony, trying to reassure him and calm him so that he wouldn't struggle too much. He invariably still managed to bite one of us. We all exchanged a look of relief if the first shot at a vein produced a sufficient blood flow, but having been tested for this and that, his veins used so many times, he was difficult to bleed.

Each subsequent puncture was a knife in my heart. Once over he would lash out at me, his little fists flaying, his hot tear-stained face a reproach. How could he understand why his mother allowed such things to happen to him? I explained to him beforehand that it would hurt, that there would be a sharp point, which he understood from previous nappy pins, and that we wanted some 'dab' (this was Anthony's word for blood).

Talking him through the experience he calmed, and when older I found this invaluable as each bleeding session became more and more difficult. The samples had to be at the laboratory in London by 11 a.m. Anthony, soothed, was passed to mother while the doctors had a cup of tea and the nurse packed the test tubes. I quickly changed my blood-smeared indoor clothes to prepare for the hasty dash to catch the 9.05 train to London, an hour's journey. I always delivered the blood samples personally to Dr James; I wasn't going to risk such a precious cargo going astray en route or on arrival at a busy general hospital. Then we waited the interminable six days for results.

We tried not to be over-optimistic, but we hoped. The disappointments followed one after another, until we never allowed ourselves to become excited anymore. Fortunately – or unfortunately – such bleeding sessions occurred about every six months. We desperately wanted a donor for Anthony, but knowing what lay ahead we were secretly relieved when tests proved incompatibility. Anthony would have to be clear of any minor infection, even an infected tooth, then be immuno-suppressed and placed in a plastic sterile bubble at the hospital.

How hard I tried to imagine my little lad in such confines, more restricted than an isolation cubicle. He had, as an aftermath of his isolation, come to resent even a closed door and we freely left all the doors in the cottage open (a slight embarrassment, in the case of the loo, to the unaccustomed visitor).

This clearance period before a transplant could' take weeks or even months. The immuno-suppression is to enable the host cells to multiply and not be rejected as foreign tissue. The crucial period is about the eighth day after the implant of donor cells, when all can go smoothly or all hell can let loose, producing reverse reactions with fatal results. Anthony would lose most of his hair and after the implant would, I knew, be sterile. This was particularly heart-breaking because I knew that if I had more children a boy would most certainly have the same condition and I couldn't face the past again, nor be instrumental in producing a little one to suffer so. And if I had a girl she would be a carrier and have to face such a decision herself when she reached womanhood.

I had one child. I felt it irresponsible to have more. I knew I would never become a grandmother. Anthony was all I had. Perhaps my critics may now understand my desperate love for Anthony and my desire to keep my son.

As the newspaper reports told the world of the latest failure of tests I was approached by Simon Welfare of Yorkshire Television for an hour-long documentary about Anthony, our way of life, Dr James and our pioneer medical project. I was keen to co-operate despite the work involved. Through the visual power of television, more than any other media, I believed I could draw attention to Anthony and others like him.

At this stage 42 other children were awaiting donors at the Westminster Hospital alone. On an average two died each week, hopelessly, without a donor, without a chance. Multiply that number by major hospitals around the world and it will indicate the demand for facilities for bone marrow transplants and relate the unrecorded death toll.

Hours and hours of filming followed, showing Anthony playing in the garden, my relating the past, my present work, my future hopes.

Film was shot of Dr James and our laboratory technicians at work, the taking of blood samples, preparing of blood clot slides for the microscope and the complex reading of reactions to produce the tissue-type of the donor. This was unpaid work by all members of our team. We thought at last our struggle was to be revealed to the world. Simon Welfare was now waiting the *piece de resistance,* the donor for Anthony and the filming of his transplant to complete the documentary. In the meantime he and his entire crew were departing for Houston in Texas to do a bit of filming of David, the boy in the bubble. David had a brother born with an immune deficiency who, like Britain's Andrew Bostic, sadly died.

When David was born, in anticipation of the same blood disorder, he was placed immediately in a sterile tent. Tests showed he was also immune deficient and as he grew, larger sterile bubbles or plastic tents were made to create his world. The funding of these tents and additional equipment, even the power supply, was by a government grant in the United States, as were his intense medical, educational and psychiatric care. Anthony received no assistance at all, yet David still needs a donor. Like Anthony, no member of his family is compatible to donate bone marrow.

As the work at the Anthony Nolan Laboratories is the only major donor testing programme, David's life revolves around the fruition of our medical project, and the compiling of a comprehensive donor register.

Marian, continuing her stalwart work, had visited a local businessman, Michael Reynolds, managing director of Spa grocery chain. She rang me with the tremendous news that they were to organise a promotion throughout their shops in Britain, raising funds by means of an own-label collection scheme. I went to London and met Michael and his public relations and advertising consultants. They guaranteed a minimum donation of £25,000.

This Spa promotion yanked the medical project to viability and solvency. The Press was sceptical about the motives of private enterprise being involved with principles such as mine. But does it really matter when the end product is to save children's lives? Max Bygraves kindly presented the cheque to Professor Humble, a senior member of the transplant team, at Selfridges Hotel in London. I tried to explain the value of the Spa promotion to Press, radio and television, but in Britain it is construed as free advertising. Yet it is an accepted form of fundraising in Australia. When a company supports a pioneer medical project, they deserve acclaim. The Spa promotion, in all, raised £31,000 and enabled us to contemplate forming our present medical and research trust and find suitable premises so our work could expand.

Dr James had a colleague at St Mary Abbotts Hospital in Kensington, London, who had mentioned that the old pathological laboratories were closed and unused. On inspection Dr James and I agreed that with vision, funding and time they could be changed to suit our needs. In addition to the salaries of technicians and the laboratory secretary I now had to provide further funds to renovate and equip the proposed Anthony Nolan Laboratories. A list of the complex equipment was compiled which I circulated to existing supporting groups and those who expressed interest. Soon items of equipment were adopted as an incentive to reach a target to enable their purchase. We all had much to do. I had to condense a year's work into a few summer months and the journeys to and from London in the heat were demanding.

Chapter 11

Summer ended abruptly with September's torrential rain, and with the rain came the dread of infection again from colds and 'flu, and the greater challenge of a third winter's isolation.

After a wonderful summer we approached it with more optimism and training. Colds usually came with a change in weather. With luck, after such a summer the usual influenza epidemic might hold off until the end of the year. Linda made preparations to return home and I began hastily planning. From Carrier's Bulk Store I purchased cartons of detergent, canned and packet foods, tinned meats and multilitres of disinfectant.

The little car chugged backwards and forwards each day, a mini freight train. I had to gauge all our requirements until spring. It was like stocking a fort. Soon it would be just three of us tucked away inside, and the world outside.

We had laboratories now being renovated; the donor testing programme was running smoothly. Although we never seemed to have sufficient funds we somehow managed to continue with unexpected generous donations. Yet I was now preparing for a third winter's isolation to keep Anthony alive. Exhausted and wet from unloading the car once again, I slumped onto a carton of disinfectant and stared at the steamy rain-spattered window, head on my palm, the epitome of Rodin's statue. I was lost in confused thoughts between the past, present and future.

Anthony would soon be four years old, double his expected life span. A miracle, or just our tremendous care? Perhaps I was preparing for this winter unnecessarily and Anthony's donor would be found, his transplant over with and he'd be home for Christmas … free, fit and well and able to lead a normal life. Tomorrow! I was always planning for tomorrow's world, but what did tomorrow hold? What if a donor wasn't found for Anthony? How long could we continue this way of life? Or if Anthony died, hopelessly, how could I continue to live without him? The rain from my wet hair trickled down my back and jolted me to return to my unloading. Shaking myself down like a shaggy old hound, I removed my wet clothes and with them that rare cloak of the doldrums, and stuck that and the containers away.

Anthony, awake from his nap now, had clambered off my bed and come to greet me. Whenever I returned from these shopping trips and re-entered the kitchen door he always looked beyond me with a look of anticipation. I knew he was looking for Linda. When he saw she wasn't with me, he would say: 'Linda's gone for a bottle of milk.' In our part of rural Kent even the milkman didn't call and the milk had to be collected by Linda from the village shop each morning. Now Anthony had exceptionally keen hearing and sense of smell. I believe this was nature's way of compensating him for his poor sight for quite a few months after his early brain surgery. He would easily hear the chinking of milk bottles as Linda turned into the driveway. He would pop his head out of the door, saying, 'There's my Linda, look.' He could tell Nanna's flip-flopping gum boots, and even before I heard her approach from the garden Anthony would be at the door with, 'There's my Nanna, look.' With the approach of my car he would be waiting, pressed so close to the door that I would need to open it carefully an inch or so at a time and call my greetings, squeeze in and whisk him high into the air for a kiss.

He needed us so desperately now. Any time we had to leave him for a few minutes or hours we would be eager to hurry back to him. We knew he would be waiting, listening. We mourned the passing of that glorious summer and its freedom. Having such a large garden we hadn't encouraged Anthony to go out onto the Lees, the large village green. Many dogs and cats roamed the area; horses cantered to and fro and at times it was even penned off for sheep to graze away the long grass. At night it moved with a sea of rabbits, and beyond it, day and night, a busy road carried pilgrims to and from beautiful Canterbury Cathedral.

Anthony had come to expect doors to be open from early morning until dusk and fits of rage followed struggles to let in the winter's blustering chill showers. He had also become used to toddling out in light cotton clothes, or none at all, and he would now tolerate only a vest and T-shirt, no pants and no shoes. Such had been his dance with nature.

He tried to stare through the rain and even attempted to run out and play, rapidly returning, teeth chattering. I had to let him do this several times. He was furious and resentful; his damp hair was rubbed in the glow of the stove and I tugged off his wet shirt.

'Switch it on, Mummy,' he cried. 'Switch it on.' I flicked on the kitchen light against the grey day. 'No! No!' he whimpered. 'The sun, Mummy, the sun!' How could I explain why the sun had gone? I tried to tell him it was winter again but the joy of summer had erased or locked away previous distressing memories. I brought out his pushchair and his clothes, but he flatly refused to dress. I couldn't cajole nor demand his co-operation; it as impossible to force Anthony to do anything, because of his condition.

Handled firmly, as a normal toddler, he would be left bruised, a pattern of fingerprints. He also had his own device to control a situation and command attention: by banging his head, he precipitated haemorrhages. Master Nolan could make me very angry by bashing his nose and plastering the blood on the walls.

Beaten into submission by a howling north-easterly, he returned to the fire and clambered on to my lap. We sang to the flames as the wind howled and the rain lashed the cottage, blotting out the sounds of summer.

Gradually we were returning to the monotony of winter isolation. Warmed by the fire, I reflected on the seasons' sounds. So used were we in isolation to nature's stirrings that the sounds of humans, a car, footsteps, or a knock proved discordant. We had few visitors in winter. The hardy, cheery postman was one of our contacts with the world. He shared a cup of tea over the top half of our barnstyle kitchen door and returned the cup with village news, which kept us a little in touch with our neighbours. Bob, short, rustically sturdy, his wild blond hair and beard tossed with the wind or snow-crusted, would appear daily with his dog Boots at heel, to be warmed on bitter winter days. His roughened hands would rim his steaming mug of tea which misted his piercing blue eyes and hid his face with its all-weather tan. Bob was a local lad with an enchanting Kent accent; he worked on the nursery behind us and had become our friend by shyly watching our efforts at hardy tasks like demolishing, sawing and carrying. Then he would leap the fence and lend a hand and barrow away the unwanted debris. I think Linda was a strong attraction, but even when Linda left he still called most days to check all was safe, to say hello to Anthony, who would kiss him through the windowpane.

Our world of green drained to shades of gold and brown. Some autumns were magnificent, the leaves crisply ablaze. But the rain had reaped a sudden change and the land was steaming. Low fogs rose as a watery sun battled ineffectively against the barrage of clouds. Leaves hung limp and wizened like flaps of aged skin torn with each sputter of the angry north-easterly as he spat them on lawn, roof and windowpane. The wind moaned at his premature calling, the drains gurgled, choked with leaves and overwork, and the trees swayed and creaked.

I disliked the cold weather as intensely as Anthony but mother preferred to be out whenever possible, clearing the garden leaves, tending her planting and borders, digging over her vegetable patch and chopping wood for the stove. I would lift Anthony onto the windowsill to watch her as she passed busily to and fro. They shouted and waved and blew kisses to each other. But I could not persuade him to go out to join her.

Then she would bustle in, leaving her mud-clogged gumboots outside, smelling richly of earth, wood-smoke, paraffin and pungent burning rotting vegetation. She would peel off her gardening clothes to step into the hot bath I had run off to steam herself to Anthony's chortles.

I now used the long dark days of winter to teach Anthony again. I used Smarties to teach him his colours, hoping he would try one. But he would plop them into my mouth, telling me the colours. I taught him to handle numbers up to 20 and we would count Smarties, windowpanes, building bricks, bottles of milk, fingers, toes … anything within our environment which I could use productively. We enriched our days with music, playing all kinds from classical, pop and ballet to the Wombles. I have taught Anthony simple dance steps and we Wombled many an hour away. One game of pivoting in circles was his special favourite; faster and faster until he became an aeroplane and I whirled him round and round, landing him gently on the settee. I know who became tired first. Anthony would say, 'Have a breather, Mummy.' Then, seconds later, he'd be tugging at my limp arm to begin again. This pivoting began every winter, triggered off like Pavlov's dogs. It had begun in Westminster Hospital in the isolation of 1973, when the only space was within the confines of the isolation cubicle, where any reasonably fast mobile game had to be in circles. Carefully guiding Anthony round and round me I tried to break this confined circle habit by running games across the lounge, round the dining room, touching a window, touching a chair, and whizzing down the long hallway to mother's bedroom; at the end I'd touch the wall and start back again. This is how I ran off his energy and tried to teach Anthony and make him happy.

He loved blowing bubbles, catching balloons, tickles, and romping. My bed became a trampoline once again, but he was drawn irresistibly back to striding round in circles. And so we revolved the time away to Anthony's fourth birthday. We would register this birthday as a special event, a celebration, so the evening before – on December 1 – we decorated the lounge and the Christmas tree, placing his birthday presents beneath it. This was the same pretty, garish silver tree I had purchased in Pimlico market, brought out now for the third time. The same now-jaded fairy was there planked on top, the same pretty lights draped round like a snake in the Palace of Minos in Crete to be flicked alive by a 20th-century switch tomorrow morning, to light a day in the life of a little boy. I checked that Anthony was snug and asleep. He lay, flushed cheek resting on his little fist, and I held my breath to listen to his sleep and gaze on his now-untroubled little face and thought of tomorrow's milestone.

Four years! In the multi-coloured glow from the fairy lights we crackled the wrapping paper and sticky tape on Anthony's many gifts ... a musical box, a tipper truck from Daddy, and a tricycle from Auntie Lily. And I opened a long-kept bottle of Scotch, originally for Christmas, and we curled by the fire, Mother and I, relaxing in the soft lounge tones.

Early on December 2, 1975, Anthony crooned the dawn chorus and our day began as I lifted my soft toddler, warm from sleep and damp from nature. Mother raked the flickering embers in the lounge fire and added more fuel as I brought Anthony to the warmth of the new flames and a new day. We sang, 'Happy Birthday to You.' 'Hip, hip hooray!' he shouted with glee. As the light improved I brought out Anthony's third birthday cake, a figure '3' carefully stored from our Manston cottage, and placed it side by side with his fourth birthday cake, a number '4' clearly emblazoned with Happy Birthday Anthony.

We revelled again in our private celebration before breakfast, of lighting the birthday candles and cheering and cheering. Four years ... a victory greater than any FA World Cup, a victory of one little fellow on this mighty globe to fight on and on and on.

We cheered, Mum and I, over our morning cup of tea and wiped away with slight embarrassment the accompanying tears of joy. The camera crews were geared for midday, the best light. It was mild and the rain held off, and opening the French windows they filmed and photographed from outside as we were inside, cheering and blowing out, only too happily, those four symbolic candles. Anthony's happy birthday was the cameras, the lights, the crewmen, the photographers ... the clicks, flashes and the 'Again

Anthony! Again, please!' just as a normal child's is a gathering of cake-eating, candy-crunching, chocolate-smudged, finger sticky contemporaries. Anthony's happiness was captured forever in those birthday photographs.

If I thought for a minute he disliked being photographed, or he objected at all, I would not have agreed, but it was attention being directed towards him and he loved it. I never allowed him to be manipulated during photography or filming sessions. They simply had to capture him *au nature!,* beaming and bathed, bare-bottomed and blotchy, as the case may be. When I could see he had tired of a session then I called a halt, and for whatever programme, journal or magazine, that was that.

My wonderful friends in the media and our unknown friends celebrated with us," witnessed by the hundreds of birthday and Christmas cards for Anthony which arrived from all parts of the globe.

* * *

Soon after Dr James returned from his trip to New Zealand he was contacted by the medical centre where he had lectured in Auckland. A Samoan Islander had the exact tissue type as Anthony. This man was Maolo Joave, a young laboratory technician. Arriving at work one day just before Christmas he was asked if he would fly to London immediately to try to save the life of a small boy. Without question, without a moment's hesitation, this burly, shy Samoan within hours was arriving at Heathrow by British Airways jet to a staggering reception of TV cameras.

He was dark and bearded and his features were astonishingly similar to Anthony's. I watched his arrival on the National News; he was to rest for 24 hours before tests. I had geared our local doctor for bleeding Anthony.

How could I have felt so positive that this time was the time? But I did! My God, how I did!

The bleeding session took place at home the next day, as distressing as usual despite our optimism at Anthony's would-be saviour arriving symbolically at Christmas time. The Simon Welfare Yorkshire TV documentary crew were on hand, having returned from America, and filmed me leaving our ice-bound cottage with the warm test-tubes of blood clutched in my gloved hand for the dash to the *9:05* to London. Only this time, bless him, one of the crew had scraped the ice off my car's windscreen and started and warmed up the engine for my hasty departure. There was a hold-up at the T-junction of the A251 on the Canterbury/ Ashwood Road and I zoomed on the outside lane, infringing all traffic regulations. I had to catch that 9:05. Another film crew boarded the train and, breathless and tense, I conducted interviews in the hour's journey to London.

On my arrival at Westminster Hospital by cab I was met by an entourage of Press and TV units from all over the world. As the taxi slowed to a halt and I saw the gathering I felt like crumbling on the floor. We may have felt alone and lost in our remote cottage, but I was wrong. I was jolted to a realisation that the world did care about the rights of one little boy. I lifted my chin, blinked back the tears and stepped out of the London cab to shake hands with this Samoan, this wonderful stranger who had crossed the world from summer to winter for the love of Anthony. As I handed over the blood samples we gave a crossed fingers sign for the world as Anthony and Maolo's blood intermingled in the laboratory labyrinths below.

I was exhausted by the TV and Press demands for interviews. All I could really concentrate on was that at this precise moment Anthony's and Maolo's blood cells were struggling in test tubes for acceptance or rejection.

In the early evening I returned to rural Kent to await the results of the six days of tests, overly optimistic and not too disturbed by our break in isolation as no influenza epidemic had struck. Those days seemed a lifetime, though I spent most of them answering press calls.

As the clock marched towards four p. m. on that sixth day and the early winter's evening drew in I was sitting in Dr James' office at Westminster Hospital. Maolo was at Marian's home in Buckinghamshire suffering with a cold; he had left New Zealand in summer in only a T-shirt to face the winter of England.

The professors called me into a separate office and told me the results of the tests. Maolo's cells had attacked Anthony's, and an implant was impossible. I calmly accepted the news but I had to pull myself together to appear before the world awaiting the results in the hospital foyer.

Yes, I did want to scream in despair. Yes, I wanted to sit in a corner and weep in private. But these were luxuries. I faced the cameras and tried to explain my disappointment. Once again I had been conducting interviews all day in anticipation of the results of the tests. To say I was exhausted is an understatement. My eyes were red-rimmed and bloodshot. It was five p.m. and I was due to appear on the Eamon Andrews TV show at six o'clock. The day had been too much. I abruptly set off for home.

It was only alone in the compartment on the evening train home that the full impact of the day's events hit me. I began to shiver, my teeth chattering uncontrollably, yet my head felt on fire. I was glad of the empty compartment as I placed my forehead on the cold windowpane and, staring at the unresponsive, flickering, multiplied moonface, moaned, 'No! Oh No!' Mother was waiting when I returned and we shared a cup of hot soup. The old stove enjoyed a frosty night and spat and roared happily up its thick black pipe. I squatted on my hands and propped my back against its warm door.

We always spoke our hearts in the kitchen. I had expected to find Mum in tears of disappointment, but she cheerily bustled round handing me more soup, a look of concern on her face. I must have looked ghastly. Mother doesn't usually fuss. She had held the fort single-handed all day, looking after Anthony and coping with the constant phone calls, and had him safely off to bed. 'Well, it's all for the best really,' she finally spoke. 'I was dreading the thought of what was ahead for Anthony, the poor little chap, going back into hospital, that isolation tent and all. It's all for the best.' She sighed again with relief, blowing the steam off her soup. This was how we reacted now, hoping desperately yet feeling a reprieve for Anthony when tests failed.

Ted was kept well informed of events, as they were reported in Australia. He'd telephone the morning of the tests and to commiserate when they failed. I didn't really feel like communicating. His powerful, hearty voice was out of tune in our world. He seemed so detached from it all I realised that at that time he did live in another world. I sensed he was not alone making that phone call and that he wouldn't be spending his Christmas alone either. Apart from a Christmas card I stopped writing.

* * *

We knew that it was very early days in the treatment of non-relative bone marrow transplants, less than three years since the medical breakthrough. Much had still to be learned, as everyone involved readily admitted. I knew that Anthony would be virtually a guinea pig. I knew that his chances of success at this stage would be 60 to 40 in his favour. I knew the trauma involved for a toddler and I also knew that it was Anthony's only chance of life.

Having Anthony with us, we knew he was at constant risk from infection, but as time passed advances were being made which would improve that 60/40 success rate. I was reluctant to hand him over yet to the doctors but desired intensely the reassurance of having his compatible donor found and on standby to make that decision.

Maolo was still quite ill and very homesick. I was able to speak to him on the telephone; he was close to tears expressing his disappointment at not having been able to help Anthony. And as mother and I once again shared our Christmas lunch alone, Maolo, the gentle giant, was seated overhead somewhere as his plane crossed Kent on the way home to New Zealand.

Chapter 12

The year 1975 clicked to 1976 ... we watched the clock hands move and toasted the New Year. Then Mum and I trundled off to our respective beds, each harbouring our secret hopes for this New Year. Simon Welfare and his Yorkshire TV documentary crew were promised the filming of the next bone marrow transplant. Everyone had been hoping it would have been Maolo and Anthony.

The next transplant scheduled was on a teenage patient, Martin Rowson, and his donor was his younger brother. This transplant was filmed. Thank God, it was a success. Martin is now fit and well, but soon afterwards Mr and Mrs Rowson learned a second son, Richard, was afflicted with the same disease. It was a big blow, after the strain of seeing Martin through his transplant. This time no family member was suitable to donate bone marrow. Sadly, he died before a compatible donor was found.

I thought this TV documentary would tell all, that it would inform those who thought their case, or that of their child's, hopeless. It would, I believed, act as a lifeline and tell the public about the value and process of tissue-typing and bone marrow transplant work and ensure that our donor register speedily came to fruition. Later, when it was screened in the summer, I was disappointed.

January was alternately cold and wet and dry and frosty, but February busily pushed it out and arrived sunny and unusually mild. Mother could work in the garden in a light sweater and even Anthony warmed in the sun's yellow rays flooding the kitchen. It was a relief to be able to fill the coal buckets without being drenched or chilled to the bone. The cottage was a joy in summer and damned hard work in winter. Our fuel bills were astronomical to heat that large timber cottage 24 hours every day, week and month of winter. Mother chopped more wood for the stove from the pile of rotted timber beams from the demolished sheds. It was a constant chore just to keep warm, but she enjoyed it. I'm sure she vented her frustration on each piece of timber beneath her flaying axe.

The first snowdrops appeared and even the green tips of daffodils; perhaps we were going to be lucky. Our winter would be over early, as it had started early. I thought it would be marvellous to have another such summer as 1975. We had no serious influenza epidemic and February continued sunny and mild.

I foolishly accepted an invitation to go to London to a lunch interview with a lady journalist from Australia. The appointment was a Saturday at the end of February, a day noticeably colder. On Monday morning I awoke, horrified. I licked the perspiration from my top lip, ran my tongue round my dry, cracked mouth and felt my burning head. I tried to lift it, heavy and hot as a steam iron, from my pillow and it lolled back. Gasping, I moaned, 'Anthony, oh Anthony! What have I done?'

I dragged my aching body out of bed, felt the icy draughts from the old window in my room, and through my feverish gaze noted the torrents of rain. I stumbled to mother's room, dizzy and disorientated, down the strangely wavering hallway. I had to act quickly. I knew I had influenza; I had granules of antibiotic on standby. They were emulsified by adding sterile water and I directed mother to prepare it for Anthony. While this was being done I phoned our doctors in Wye. As soon as Anthony awoke I gave him a ten-mil dose of antibiotic and within minutes the doctor had arrived.

Sure enough, my greatest fears were realised. Anthony was feverish and running a temperature. I had brought influenza into the house. The doctor alerted the nearest major hospital, the Kent and Canterbury 11 miles away and called an ambulance. Anthony received emergency treatment, was placed in an isolation cubicle and put on a speedy antibiotic drip. Mother stayed at the hospital. Later, when she arrived home, she discovered me semi delirious, in a sea of perspiration, tossing about my bed and muttering, 'I've killed Anthony. I've killed him. I have! I have!'

Anthony's temperature soared to over 103 degrees. Mother sat by my bed, having once again phoned the hospital for news. It was past midnight. Sister said she would phone us if we were needed. There was nothing more we could do. Our kind doctor brought my drugs and left them, with instructions, on the kitchen table. I gulped the tablets and stared at Mum. This was the worst crisis since Anthony's brain haemorrhage four years ago and we couldn't be with him.

The doctors had expressed concern that mother might also have contacted influenza. Until this was determined it was best she kept clear of the intensive care unit. Sure enough, next morning she was aching and feverish; a massive influenza epidemic was now sweeping Britain.

At dawn I phoned the hospital. Anthony was critically ill, his fever raging. I could visualise my little boy alone in his cot calling for us fruitlessly. He would believe we had deserted him. The telephone was our only link with Anthony and the next 24 hours was absolute hell.

I recriminated myself intensely. I cursed myself to damnation. I literally beat my head, tore my hair, in my frantic ravings; a confused mixture of my raging temperature, my terror at losing Anthony, and being responsible so directly for yet more of his suffering. The telephone stirred me from a fretful doze of distressing memories. Trying to control a persistent cough I lifted the receiver and heard through my raspy breathing that Anthony had developed pneumonia; Sister said she would keep us informed. I was still numbly holding the now-useless receiver after the click and whirr down the line. Slowly I replaced it and stayed in the chair, pulling my robe around me, my head bowed on my tucked-up knees, alternately coughing and choking with tears until I seemed all swollen, throat, nose and eyes, a molten mobile emotion turned inside-out, like those faces painted by Francis Bacon, or a face distorted and reflected in moving water. After a time I straightened my stiffened limbs and, bent double, added coals to the fire and shuffled back to bed. Somehow the news leaked out of Anthony's crisis and hospitalisation. The well-meaning Press and public called all day until my burning throat could barely whisper replies. Climbing in and out of bed twisted each aching bone and lathered me in perspiration. Yet, I couldn't disconnect the phone. I was awaiting desperately each hospital bulletin. Anthony was on the critical list. Each time the phone rang and I stumbled towards it my hand hesitated a fraction as the lightning thought crossed my mind ... 'I'm sorry, Anthony is dead.' Between the Press calls Sister phoned; Anthony's temperature was down to 102, then 101, then 100, until it stabilised a little in the high 90s. The second crisis was over for the moment. Yet more were to follow.

Our main task in the cottage was keeping warm. Challock village, being so high above sea level, is always cold and has more snow than the surrounding valleys. Winter had returned with a vengeance as snowdrifts blocked the doors and painted each window-pane fluffy white. Ice formed on the inside of the glass, as icy-cold and sharp as the pain of my guilt, and the cottage cowered miserably against the blast, as if purposeless, lost without Anthony.

Mother and I were like two hags dragging the coal into the cottage, fighting and floundering for breath, back into the warmth inside ... two ghostly figures, black silhouettes against the orange square of the open stove door, clawing the flickering embers, frantically raking and feeding the old stove to keep warm. Cartons of canned soups were our mainstay. Clutching unsteadily a mug of soup and a refilled hot water bottle we would slowly move back to our beds.

Anthony, thank God, was still stable though weak. We shuffled through each day in the bone-racking cold, aching to be with our little boy. A week later Anthony's temperature had soared again. He had contracted diarrhoea. As I replaced the receiver I thought, 'He's so frail, he's so weak from influenza. How can his tiny body battle this? He's always known we were fighting with him. Will he give in without us beside him?' I could see him alone in his suffering and it was agony. Again the nightmare of waiting for news, the interminable days, the frustration of being unable to go to the hospital. When I drifted from one fitful sleep to another I could hear him crying, calling me. Mother's fever and the aches of 'flu abated. Before the end of two weeks she was able to go to the hospital.

Miraculously, Anthony was alive. Barely alive. Mother, pale and still weak, dressed with determination and trekked through the deep snow across the Lees to the road to Canterbury and hailed the bus. She stayed all day, returning well after dark, cold, drawn and tired. I hobbled about keeping the fires stoked, and warmed the soup, having it ready for her return. Shaking the snow from her scarf and her caked boots, I saw she was crying. The scene she described I could see in minute detail: it had all happened again.

'Anthony,' she said, 'is grey and skeletal, so weak he cannot even sit up or lift his head from his pillow. He is on an intravenous drip and convulsed with diarrhoea.' As she entered his room she had quietly said, 'Where is my baby?' He had turned his eyes in her direction and, faintly smiling, whispered, 'There's my Nanna, look.' Releasing the cot side, she stroked his head and held the thin, limp little hand in hers and for hours sang all their favourite songs. Quietly, on and on, talking to him, willing him to live, until he slept. I choked into my pillow again and again that it was all my fault. I had put the Appeal, the publicity of an interview, before Anthony. Divided loyalties. Yet they were, in a way, one and the same thing. I had done this before but had been lucky.

I prayed and prayed, fighting for breath between the persistent bouts of coughing. Dear Lord, you can't mean Anthony to die this way. He can't die without me. If he dies, so do I ... I have no life without my Anthony.

Early the next morning our GP called as mother was busily preparing to catch the early bus to Canterbury. He was baffled at my condition. The influenza should be under control by now with the antibiotics he had prescribed, but I still had a high temperature, my lungs sounded like old bellows and I had a cough that shook me like rattling a tin of nails. He diagnosed chronic bronchitis and told me strictly to stay in bed and prescribed new drugs. I really felt as if I was dying and I didn't care.

All I could think of was Anthony. Mother had said that she would be better staying at the hospital with Anthony constantly, if we were to have any hope of pulling him through in his present critical condition. I asked my doctor if he could arrange this and, to my relief, he walked to the phone and arranged with the hospital for mother to be admitted to the resident mothers' unit.

Wonderful Mother. Anthony had his Nanna; he was not alone anymore, and I was reassured all was well. As I babbled and coughed and the bed tipped and the objects in the room advanced and receded and revolved, the doctor's prescription lay untouched on the kitchen table. Awoken the next day by a persistent heavy knock on the door, I stumbled through the chill rooms to the kitchen. A neighbour had brought the milk, which had been left uncollected for three days at the village shop. The kind lady who usually brought it also had influenza.

As the news was publicised, Bob called and ensured the delivery of wood to light the fires or milk from the shop. Later, when I was able to fend a little more for myself, I would phone my orders through to the Post Office; dear Mr Puckstead of the village shop, during lunch or after the shop closed, and despite the inaccessibility through the thick snow, would bring my groceries to the door.

Mother phoned each evening with news of Anthony. The diarrhoea was easing, he could sit up, he was still on an intravenous drip, and too frail to nurse. I eagerly awaited that call each evening. I longed to be with Anthony, but I still showed no signs of improvement. I lost weight rapidly as if I had to suffer more, if possible, than Anthony.

I just couldn't get better. I found myself wandering from each empty room to another calling Anthony's name. Standing in his room I stared at his empty, stripped cot and then at the wall pasted with the hundreds of cut-outs of cats, dogs, ducks, purple elephants, gaily-waving toddlers in party hats, all cheering on the birthday number 4. We had decorated one wall in Anthony's room in the Manston Cottage with the cards from his third birthday and had done the same in his new bedroom, so that he could see from his cot lots of pretty, coloured shapes. Mother had made him a paper merry-go-round revolving beneath the light; horses, rabbits, and lions dancing on air in reflected glory when the light was switched on. We always left this dim light on all night for Anthony. He had become used to it in hospital. I switched on the light revealing the now too-tidy, empty room and flickering to life the paper animals. Would that I could bring Anthony back with such ease.

My Anthony. Oh, my Anthony, I whispered. Please God, don't let him die. I was desperate to be with him. My misery and frustration were destroying me, burning me out. After four weeks Anthony's diarrhoea had cleared. He was taken off a drip and could be nursed by his Nanna again ... a grey emaciated little figure. He was put on a new oral antibiotic. That evening mother's call held a new tone of eagerness; Anthony had eaten some baby rice. The next morning he had eaten a full bowl and during the day more and more. This was his first step towards recovery.

Mother had saved him. The hospital was wonderful, of course, but I mean the spirit, the feeling of being loved and wanted, the caring which makes the difference between a life worth living or not: From then on his appetite was voracious; baby foods were carefully prepared for him, with broths and cereals, and later stewed fruit. In five weeks I heard mother's proud yet incredulous voice saying, 'And today he even ate a whole mashed banana.' The next morning when she went just after seven o'clock to give him his breakfast she found him sitting on the floor, having rifled his locker. He had discarded the cans of baby food (one with teeth marks on it) and was clutching, with some difficulty, a huge cereal packet and tucking into it ravenously.

I raked the fire and put the kettle on, whispering 'He's eating' ... louder and louder until I was yelling to the empty cottage, 'Can you hear me? He's eating!' I found myself enjoying things I had been unable to do for years. I played dual games of scrabble curled on the sofa before a now friendly and not so demanding fire; and the creaks and sighs of the cottage were no longer ominous but comforting. I sighed in the relaxation and sheer enjoyment of being able to listen uninterrupted to the music of Schubert, Chopin, Wagner, Handel and my favourite ballet Delibes' *Coppelia*.

For years I simply hadn't had the time to spend the hours, as I did now in my convalescence, to enjoy with such abandonment all the pleasures of poetry, music and the odd zany TV programme. Now, too weak to feel guilty, I eagerly read, listened and looked.

The next week Anthony continued to improve and so did I. By the weekend I was able to see him. The kind chap from the Challock garage started up my old Anglia and I carefully drove the road to Canterbury. The snow had almost cleared, but it felt strange leaving the cottage, stepping out into the world again.

I had been bedridden for six weeks. Six whole weeks! Astounding! I had rarely been ill in my life. I felt as much of an adventurer leaving the cottage and taking off in my car as the men walking on the moon. Between the dual beauty of a blazing sunset and a rising bluish-yellow moon, thin as a wafer, the road wound down to Canterbury through orchards laid barren for the future fruit season by February's trickery. I thought how close I had come to losing the fruit of my being.

I reflected that if I felt so strange after six weeks' illness and solitude, how much worse Anthony must have felt after his months of illness from birth, and even longer isolation in the Westminster Children's Hospital. It must be as traumatic as being born over and over again; he was adjusting, ever adjusting.

I knew I couldn't go into Anthony's cubicle as I still had the residue of lung congestion and bronchitis, but I was able to see him through the glass between the curtains, without him seeing me. He was happily playing on his Nanna's lap. I don't know exactly what I expected to see from mother's reports, but I still bit my lip to hold back the tears at the sight of my frail little lad within. What must he have looked like when mother arrived five weeks ago? I silently applauded her courage.

It was another week before I could enter his cubicle. He looked and looked away and huddled closer to Nanna. He wouldn't let me hold him. I spoke quietly to him each day, sang our songs and, little by little, he allowed me to just touch him. I understood. He was blaming me. I had deserted him. All adults left him eventually … his Daddy, his Linda and then his Mummy. Only Nanna was there. Linda had been similarly severely afflicted with influenza and bronchitis, but at the end of Anthony's seven weeks she returned to the cottage and we went together to see him.

We entered the cubicle and crooned a little song we three sang in the garden the previous summer. He opened his thin little arms, encompassing our heads, and placed his head on ours. 'Lindama,' he whispered. We were forgiven.

After two months Anthony could finally come home. His departure from hospital was filmed by national television as matron and staff waved him off. They, mother and God had performed a miracle. His family, mother, Linda and I, gathered about him as he stared around the cottage once again. I gently picked him up and cradled him like a baby. He was so tiny and looking at the drawn face so little changed from my first gaze over four years ago, I reflected that our worst fears had not materialised; our baby had survived. He had survived! I very gently spun him round like an aeroplane, like the times before his illness, and he clutched me and laughed, a smile worth the world.

* * *

I dealt with the press calls and Linda was at hand to nurse and play with Anthony. Again we worked together, pouring out our love to Anthony and calming him through his nightmares when he would awake screaming and calling for us. Gradually he settled into his home again, but he wouldn't be left for a second. He had to keep one of us in his sight; he was watching, always alert, in case we disappeared, leaving him alone. The end of April was still cool with the usual flurrying showers and alternate bursts of sunshine; the garden's brown was now dappled with the yellow of daffodils, purple and white crocuses and the new greens of spring, but the blossom buds were gone, killed by the mock spring which had almost killed my son.

Following the publicity of Anthony's illness, I was contacted by Julia Morley, of Mecca Ltd, director of the Miss World Contest. Her attention had been drawn to Anthony and our medical project and she expressed an earnest desire to help. I was invited to the Carl Allen Awards at the Lyceum Ballroom, Aldwych, presented by the Duchess of Kent. There I was able to speak with Julia and her husband, Eric. It was arranged that a charity cabaret would be organised in Jersey, in the Channel Islands, by Julia and her friends to raise money for the Appeal. We were to be guests of Sir Billy and Lady Budin. Miss World was also to be a guest at the dinner, along with the star entertainers Frankie Vaughan and the comedian Freddie Davis.

I found myself on one of the tiny planes that commute from Heathrow to the Channel Islands, seated beside Frankie Vaughan. I had idolised Frankie as a teenager, with his tipped top hat and cane and leg-kicking songs ... 'Green Door,' and 'Give Me the Moonlight'. But the mature Frankie, now newly a grandfather and proud of it, was warm, relaxed and stunningly attractive. He sported a super tan, in contrast to my paleness, and emanated tremendous vitality (due, I found later, to a regular sauna and even more, I believe, to being a contented family man). He didn't really know why he was on his way to Jersey; of course, he knew the Butlins well, and I had time to explain before he spotted Freddie 'Parrot-face' Davis seated at the other end of the small plane.

They had been called to perform for charity and they had responded spontaneously. Members of the Variety Club International do such tremendous work for charity; Frankie, I knew, had for years supported boys' clubs throughout Britain. On our arrival we were shown around Sir Billy and Lady Sheila's home, a magnificent stone house with an impressive indoor swimming pool over which grapes grew m summer.

Jersey is a beautiful island with a superb climate. I already knew it well from a summer vacation many years previously, camping with my kid brother. We had walked to each of the sweeping crescents of fine sandy beaches as I taught him Chaucer and in return he taught me to appreciate sculpture. The evening was a tremendous success and raised over £3,000. This was the early days of the work done by Eric and Julia Morley through Variety Club International. Later donations from proceeds of the Miss World Beauty Contest enabled Dr James to help plan, design and purchase a multi-thousand-pound computerised tissue-typing microscope. This microscope will ensure our donor testing programme accelerates by testing blood samples automatically.

* * *

Just as automatically our lives slotted back into the same routine; days spent with Anthony, evenings in my all-purpose room answering and writing letters. Mother and I now took it in turns to cover Appeal duties. Usually I gave talks, lectures and attended the more official cheque presentations and mother enjoyed attending dances, balls and summer fetes. Once again, as the land warmed to the buzz of honeybees, a hive of wonderful supporters were on the move, busily fundraising from John o' Groats to Land's End.

Dr James and I had to meet often in London regarding the development of the laboratories, which were being equipped and renovated in stages. We needed the freedom to make decisions and implement them speedily if lives were to be saved, which necessitated forming the present medical and research trust. This involved the appointing of the Midland Bank Trust Company to act on our behalf and the appointing of Trust solicitors and accountants, and the drafting of the Trust Deed, all resolved at long meetings in Pall Mall. With the guidance and expertise of our present Committee our Trust was established.

* * *

We awaited a second blazing summer in vain. But we were happy, our days always busy. Mother restored her garden to perfection after the ravages of winter. Linda, joined by her friend Beverley, romped with Anthony, and when confined indoors I continued to teach him. Now four-and-a-half years old, he was still physically a toddler but bright and eager to learn. He still had setbacks from the ghastly haemorrhaging phases and had, unfortunately, reverted to a fixed diet of Weetabix, milk and honey, or toast and Bovril. I expressed my concern to the transplant team of doctors, yet no action was taken.

I never again met Anthony's paediatrician at Westminster Children's Hospital, after a time in 1973 when he had told me to get off the ward. He never requested to see Anthony, nor did he contact me regarding his condition. When he retired at the end of 1976, Anthony then had a sympathetic paediatrician whom I was to meet under dramatic circumstances.

Chapter 13

As my letters to Ted were infrequent and basically contained reports on Anthony, he may have come to the realisation that I felt he had failed us, especially Anthony, who more than the average child needed a father's love and attention. Perhaps I resented his freedom, leading the life of a single man and avoiding the responsibilities of being a parent. He had phoned a couple of times while I was in London organising the formation of our Medical Trust. It was unusual for me not to be at home.

I received a letter in June saying that he wanted to return for good. I had mixed feelings. In all honesty, I did not want him back again, but Anthony loved and needed his father.

Ted had been gone another 14 months. This time I didn't drive to Heathrow Airport to meet him, but just the nine miles to Ashford Railway Station. During the constrained conversation, I urged the old car up the steep gradient to Challock and I was thinking, 'You have to try to restore this crumbling relationship. He is here, so he must care. And he is Anthony's father, and Anthony needs him.'

Alone that first evening after so long, Ted circled me and, with wry amusement, commented on my pallor and said I felt spongy. It was humiliating. I knew what I looked like and under such scrutiny I felt like a discarded possession, no longer pleasurable. He could see my hurt expression and with excessive gusto roared how he liked his women plump.

But the first day was pleasant enough, and the second, as the novelty of the cottage and Anthony occupied Ted. On the morning of the third day Ted awoke coughing, sneezing and feverish. It was July in England – summer. But it was winter in Australia. He had contracted influenza on the flight over. I could think only of Anthony … we had restored him to health in the past few weeks;

his nightmares had ceased, he'd eagerly clambered into bed with his Daddy the previous two mornings.

No, please God, No. We can't go through it again, I prayed. I called our GP and he speedily alerted the hospital once again in Canterbury.

As I anxiously nursed Anthony, mother packed his cup and dish and favourite toys. I planned to drive him myself. I could stay with him this time. As we were about to leave Ted rolled over and asked mother if she could put clean sheets on the bed, as he was sweating. I can't repeat her answer.

I had Mum with Anthony seated on her lap safely in the car as the doctor arrived to see Ted. I hastily said goodbye and Ted nonchalantly peeled off his wristwatch and said, 'As you're going to Canterbury, drop this off at the jeweller's; it's losing time.' I turned my back in disgust.

I drove rapidly to the hospital and glanced at my son and remembered my own recriminations just a few months previously. A watch! A damn watch! As if I was going to have time, or feel inclined, to roam Canterbury for watch repairers when Anthony could suffer again those weeks in the spring.

Anthony was kept in hospital while Ted recovered from influenza. Thank God, Anthony miraculously did not contract it. Each day, Hugh, our new Press man for the Appeal, phoned for news of Anthony's progress. It was his job to issue daily reports on Anthony's condition.

Just before Anthony was allowed out of hospital, letters began arriving from Australia for Ted, and in his usual blasé fashion he let me read the first one, which was mainly about the transference of his driver's licence. The others arriving daily he withheld. He told me they were from a friend and work colleague who had been kind and helpful. I have always deeply respected the privacy of the individual, but with my baby once again in hospital and a Ted I did not recognise beside me, I intercepted the next letter.

It was a love letter. I had noted the carefully ironed shirts and the neatly packed suitcase on his arrival. I wasn't angry but I was curious. I wanted him to be truthful and frank about the girl but he was falsely jovial and evasive.

Mother, Linda and I knew what to expect when Anthony returned from hospital … the resurrecting of all his past fears, the demands for attention, the nightmares and the sleepless nights. But Ted saw our soothing of a distraught child, also confused by the return of his Daddy, as pandering. Anthony regularly threw his cup of Ribena at the wall and smashed his plate of toast on the hearth.

Ted picked him up and, yelling at him, slung him into his cot. I didn't object too much to this, but I could hear Ted aggressively demanding, 'Lie down! Lie down when I tell you to!' I have similarly placed Anthony in his cot when he became unmanageable but left him to get over his tantrum. And when it was all over he would say, 'Be a good boy now, Mummy,' and I would lift him out. But Anthony was just as strong-willed as his father and stood up each time Ted tried to force his head onto the pillow. Somehow Anthony managed to clamber up and bash his face brutally on the wooden edge of his cot, striking directly on the bridge of his nose. The force of the blow resulted in a fountain of blood.

I'd heard enough. I entered Anthony's room as Ted said, 'Take the child from me before I throw him through the window!' I knew Ted's anger calmed as quickly as it erupted and these were isolated incidents, but the next day Ted calmly packed his bag and left.

I wasn't sorry. It was a stranger who had left my home. Ted wanted me as I had been … a career woman, a social success, bright, attractive, adventurous and fun-loving; not what I had become – a mother with a sick baby, thin, tired, serious, dedicated to Anthony and a pioneer medical project. All this I could understand and accept, but not the deceit.

I would have preferred him to have written and said he didn't want to return, been frank so that Anthony could have been spared the distress of his daddy simply disappearing again. And I could have felt free, perhaps, to have re-married and provided Anthony with a real father, not a part-time one. After he left more letters arrived from his mistress in Adelaide.

Linda and mother were bitter in their condemnation, but I could not fan flames of anger for a dead love. I just felt deeply sorry that I had failed in a relationship so important for Anthony.

The next two weeks I cancelled appointments as Anthony was extremely disturbed. Hugh covered some for me, but the work had to go on. Our new letterheads and leaflets had to be designed and new material agreed for a promotion by Bishop Foodstores for the Appeal. Hugh kindly brought the material down from London.

Mother was in the garden. Hugh and I were working through mounds of proofs when in walked Ted. I wasn't even disturbed. I looked and simply said, 'I thought you had gone back to Australia.' A disgusting scene followed and Hugh left.

Ted had simply assumed he could walk in and out of my life without question. I had come to the end of the road. I told him I regretted the day I ever set eyes on him and, as far as I was concerned, the only good I had achieved in our relationship was encouraging his vasectomy so that he could not produce more children. He accused me of having an affair with Hugh. It was, of course, an excuse to leave without conscience. He had obviously sensed my animosity despite my previous attempts to mask it.

I thought I would do anything for Anthony. But I could not tolerate the further indignity of the relationship with his father. He left, and eventually returned to Adelaide.

Later that year of 1976 Hugh asked me to marry him. He was quite frank. He wanted me, but he didn't want Anthony. I believe it was then I realised that I never wanted to re-marry. The demands were too much, the emotional scars of past relationships too deep. I found the domestic subservient role rancid, so I spat it out, shook my mane and steered again to my goal of Anthony and all he represents. I closed a part of me, the part responding as a woman. I de-personalised ... *I* did not exist anymore. I had lost me, Shirley, somewhere along the line. I no longer desired anything for myself, no longer resented my constant care of Anthony or the demands of the Appeal. I was a mother and campaign leader. Nothing else was important.

At times, I had almost accepted invitations to go out with attractive men. At times I was very, very lonely and at times felt I could not cope much longer with Anthony and the ever-growing web of responsibility of our rapidly expanding laboratory project, which was demanding more and more support. I reached a stage when, at the end of each day, I tried to close my eyes and rest, but my fears for Anthony, tomorrow's duties, and the full weight of my responsibilities, left me frantically tossing and turning my head, so I took more sleeping tablets, and more and more! It was the only way I could switch off to cope with another day, and I did cope with other days. I had closed the door on the past.

* * *

The fundraising continued and it was especially heart-warming to feel the kind support of so many people still battling along with me for Anthony's life. The daily letters of love and encouragement were, and still are, a tremendous help.

The time came for the screening of the documentary by Simon Welfare of Yorkshire Television. Now I was sure our struggle and the deplorable plight of children like Anthony would be revealed to the world. It was called 'The Boy in the Bubble.' I watched the first half, a fascinating filming about David in Houston, Texas, living in two large sterile bubbles constructed in the lounge of his parents' enormous American home. A moving and articulate account of David's daily routine was given by his mother, stunningly beautiful and immaculately groomed; calm and unharassed. Accounts were given of David's progress by his group of psychiatrists, doctors and professors and his private tutor, calling daily at the home. The film showed his sterile mobile unit to transfer him to a specially constructed sterile playroom for observation in hospital, and finally a miniature spacesuit at a cost of thousands of dollars so that he could walk in the outside world. At last, the latter part of the film showed Dr James and our technicians at work tissue-typing donor blood samples, then the cameras moved to the list of critical patients on the laboratory wall. Their names and tissue-type clearly displayed, David's and Anthony's at the top. The film showed Martin's transplant and his recovery, and others at the Westminster Children's Hospital.

Then came film of Anthony in his simulated isolation within the confines of our cottage and a short interview with me stating how my work must continue. It was not stated in the film that all the work in Britain was solely dependent upon charity. It was not stated that David's life, like Anthony's, depended on my efforts to raise money and the resulting public support to enable Dr James and his staff to continue their vital work. It was guaranteed David would stay alive in his specially created sterile world provided by an American Government grant.

In Britain, on the other hand, children like David and Anthony were dying each week. No such Government grants were provided to keep *them* alive. Anthony was alive only by our love, care, chance and God's design. I was driving myself into the ground to fund a world register of donors, yet the funding of David's spacesuit cost more than our annual running costs. I know that the immediate question that springs to mind is why the United States was not funding a donor register such as ours. The fact is the need there is not as imperative as in Europe. Hundreds of successful bone marrow transplants have been performed in the United States, especially in Seattle, but as the birth ratio is an average of four children to a family, inevitably one child in the family proves suitable to donate bone marrow.

In Europe, with no population increase and two children to a family, the need is greater for non-relative donors. I wonder to this day if David's mother is aware that her son's life lies mainly with the success or failure of the Anthony Nolan Laboratories? Certainly the documentary gave no indication of this. David is still alive at the time of writing and still in isolation; he is well-balanced, normally developed, articulate and literate.

Anthony is out of isolation, under-formed, seriously disturbed, has suffered a nervous breakdown and developmentally is three years of age. The psychiatrist and educational help I sought so desperately for him in Britain never happened. He has been deprived medically, psychologically, socially and educationally. I was bitterly disappointed with the documentary, for which we had all worked so hard, especially British doctors and professors.

There were many other news and TV reporters, however, who reported dynamically after interviews. Linda Lee Potter, of the London *Daily Mail*, presented several excellent articles generating support and fearlessly attacking government apathy and misdirected priorities and wasted expenditure. She is. a busy mother as well as a journalist whose style reflects the humanist and the intellectual. She swings from wholesome rib-tickling family humour to satire or accurate gut-kicking criticism.

Linda's notes were scribbled rapidly over lunches at Stone's Chop House in London, where I was privileged to enjoy her company as well as the excellent cuisine. To our amazement we discovered we had had the same tutors at drama school. Linda's articles generated a flood of response from male readers. She wrote of our target of £50,000 needed to provide a Zeiss computerised microscope. A cheque for £1,000 was sent to me by Mr Churchill from Cumbria and he wrote to the *Daily Mail* urging 50 others who could afford it to do the same. A widower in his 70s who'd followed my work since its inception, he wrote to me sadly disappointed when his suggestion was not publicised. But this did not negate his spontaneous gesture of love and friendship for a little boy he had never met. I was to meet Mr Churchill months later as we shared a day in Canterbury and a prayer in the beautiful cathedral.

Frankie McGowan and Charles Langley of the London *Evening News* were also responsible for positive, detailed reporting. Frankie, a mother with two young children, related directly and personally to Anthony's story. She came down to the cottage and was able to meet him and see the ravages of his disease and isolation. John Snow of ITN, Alan Hargreaves, Barry Westwood and his Southern TV crew, all continued their excellent reports, as did the 'Today' programme, Radio London, BBC Radio and Pebble Mill and the Australian media.

Calls from Australia were frequent, and because of the time difference, at an unsociable hour, usually after midnight. Aching to crawl into bed, curled up in my armchair awaiting my cue, it was not unusual to be broadcasting live, just about, bouncing 12,000 miles by satellite on to a breezy breakfast show. Mother, teacher and playmate by day ... secretary, politician and news-speak by night.

Such qualifications were called on to deal with a crisis which almost destroyed years of work.

A Westminster Hospital administrator interpreted a new directive by the Department of the Environment to read that all employees must be on two-year contracts and their employers – in our case the Anthony Nolan Appeal – had to have two years' salaries in advance. The previous ruling with hospital administrations had been one year in advance. For example, before we could employ or even advertise for our first technician it was necessary to raise the $5,000 to cover the annual salary. Now, with a staff of six, it would mean having over $100,000 in advance. It was not possible. We barely managed to keep ahead of our running costs and still had no government assistance, yet during Britain's worst economic recession we had managed to survive so far by the will of the people.

I had to fight for one of our important technicians and our laboratory secretary who handled all the donor sessions, computer printouts, donor searches for patients, the organisation of compatibility tests and the busy day-to-day inquiries. Both were now threatened with the sack. Hugh, our information director, contacted friends in the press and the interpretation of the Act became a national issue. Primarily I was battling to keep staff without whom our project could not continue.

Representatives of the Department of the Environment were interviewed, MPs invited on to TV programmes. As I put my point and they theirs, it was mayhem. Everyone appeared to interpret the Act as they desired without regard to the consequences. I simply wanted the work of the laboratories to continue uninterrupted. The Act apparently was to create job security.

The Department of the Environment said that the hospital administration had misinterpreted the Act, but the hospital administration refused to alter their policy. Such adamant policy had retired Betty, our previous laboratory secretary – active and highly competent – on the dot of her retiring age of 60. After numerous hours of interviewing applicants in London I had found David Bedford as a replacement. Now David's job as a dedicated member of our team was threatened by bureaucracy. David, who never left the laboratory till well after normal office hours, put in hours of voluntary overtime.

No, I would not accept it. This was a worrying time for David, having left a secure job for the past 10 years with a foreign embassy. I asked him quietly to have confidence in me and he worked on. I was not going to let this project die, Act or no Act, hospital administration or not. Meetings and controversy, hostility and resentment by the hospital administration followed the publicity, but *they* had started the battle by firing the first shot.

I was expected to accept the dismissals of our office and laboratory staff without question, and in turn the severing of Anthony's only lifeline. I returned volley for volley. The result was a rallying of volunteers on my side of the battle and the people won the day by raising sufficient money to cover the administration's requirements of two years' salaries in advance. We saved our staff, but people in high places were irate and felt their authority was questioned, irrespective of principle or truth. Pride can be, unwittingly, disastrously destructive. Uncomfortable working relations within a hospital complex are not conducive to progress and our medical team suffered greatly. Ruffled feathers had to be smoothed!

Politically, we reached a 'Catch 22' situation of chasing our tail and Hansard reported the official Government line ... 'The success rate is not high enough to warrant Government backing ... more transplants need to be carried out to produce evidence of the efficacy of the treatment.'

'How the hell can we do more transplants,' I yelled at the cottage walls, 'if we don't have the bloody donors? My son will be a guinea pig to aid medical science. I accept this because there is a chance, his only chance, that he may just come through alive and be cured. Yet the Department of Health will not even accept the sacrifice of my only son.'

I was torturing myself in anger and frustration, pacing the room, muttering and alternatively retrieving Hansard and flinging it back at the walls. A round-table conference was eventually arranged with the Minister of Health, his advisers, the full transplant team and myself for December 13. I awaited the meeting with anticipation, not optimism. In the meantime the complex laboratory work continued, guided by the expertise of Dr James, who pushed himself to the limits as a busy director of the blood transfusion service of Westminster Hospital as well as the driving force behind our donor register programme. He worked many hours in a voluntary capacity to train and supervise staff and design and equip the Anthony Nolan Laboratories. There were times when we were able to work together, enjoyably and productively, such as when we were invited to lecture to doctors and friends of the European community in Luxembourg. Couples of all nationalities came to support our work financially and personally wish us well. The Luxembourg visit pleasurably stopped us in our serious tracks. Cynthia Albrecht, our hostess, and her friends continue to support our work.

Chapter 14

With incredulity I ordered Anthony's birthday cake in the shape of the numeral 5. The staff of Knevett's Bakery in Ashford again made and presented Anthony with a magnificent cake. We made the same preparations ... the silver Christmas tree, the lights, the gifts and the cameras set to record the event; the same lonely birthday of a little boy cheering as he blew out his candles, his party friends – the film crews – at a safe distance through the French windows, cheering with him. I destroyed the old figure 4 cake, flinging it into the bin. The fifth would soon be stored away; like Anthony, I thought, to be produced each year for the cameras. So I cheered with him, the baring of my teeth and my masked smile just a little short of a scream. Five years! Five years! echoing down into the well of my self-control. Why can't he be free? Damn the Government! Damn all the power-polling, insincere, faceless ones spouting democracy.

Abraham Lincoln said: 'Government *OF* the people, *FOR* the people, *BY* the people.' And as George Bernard Shaw replied, not with such an exact expletive: 'Balls!' A word I would liked to have used at the meeting on December 13, 1976, at the Department of Health in London.

The Health Minister was unavoidably detained. His Under-Secretary, Eric Deakins, was his surprisingly young, friendly and sympathetic, if somewhat nervous, representative. ITN were allowed to film the gathering round the huge oval table; later a film of Anthony and myself at home was added; with the comments offered by MP Keith Speed outside after the meeting. Eric Deakins and Keith Speed began the discussion; the Minister's advisers – male and female – gave their views. Their adversaries were some of the world's leading professors, immunologists, pathologists, doctors and paediatricians, and, in my humble position, a mother, who somehow had kept a little boy alive for five years despite his medical condition.

As a result of that meeting, almost a year later, the transplant team did receive an annual grant for research of £18,000 for three years. The donor testing programme, this scratch on the surface of progress, at least was better than nothing at all.

I realised that barely three years had passed since Simon Bostic's transplant and that I was trying to keep one step behind a breakthrough in medical science. Decades usually pass before treatment becomes universally available. I can remember the screening for tuberculosis at school ... even watching an uncle die from it. Then it was a voracious killer. Now it's easily curable like many other diseases. I do think of the years of dedicated work to beat these killer diseases of earlier years and the millions who died while doctors battled ignorance, fear, professional jealousy and scepticism. I had not realistically anticipated a great deal from the Ministry of Health meeting and, in consequence, was not unduly disappointed by the outcome.

Taking small steps is better than not being able to walk at all. We had a foot in the door. They could no longer pretend we did not exist.

The new transplant paediatrician at the meeting of the Department of Health watched the national news that evening. He saw the section of the film on Anthony and contacted me the next day, saying he wished to see my son. He came to our cottage, rather than risk bringing Anthony to London.

Our second meeting confirmed my first impressions ... that of an extremely competent doctor and a kind, concerned man when dealing with a distraught child. He had to take blood samples and I assisted. This doctor was quite frank, which I appreciated. He feared that Anthony had been kept on steroid drugs for too long. His appearance on television had prompted his concern.

Anthony had grown barely an inch in three years; his face was large, round and puffy, his square shoulders tapered to thin, underformed legs. The specialist's fear was that such continued exposure to the drug prednisolone had destroyed vital glands which Anthony would need to function when immuno-suppressed during a bone marrow transplant. Without this he could not possibly tolerate, let alone survive, a transplant.

It had taken three years before Anthony· could officially be released from the paediatrician who had treated him after arrival in Britain in 1973. He had now retired. His new paediatrician, an expert accurately discussing Anthony's disease with me, knew I understood what he was saying. 'We have to begin with a withdrawal programme,' he said. 'We must reduce Anthony's daily steroid dosage each week, month by month, and hope its damaging effects are not irreparable.' He left to drive the 60 miles back to London, clutching the tubes of Anthony's blood, concern in his face. I closed the door against the winter and, leaning back on its ridged wood, I felt unquestioned confidence in Anthony's new man. I also felt a shiver of fear – if Anthony's glands had been destroyed, then his case was now quite hopeless.

Why had he been kept on steroids for so long? Why had it never been questioned?

I had now to strictly record the drug dosages and mark off the periods when they were reduced. I was also asked to submit three-monthly reports to the transplant paediatrician in London.

* * *

A few days before Christmas, 1976, sitting in my room, a feeling of disaster overwhelmed me. The night was oppressively silent, as if the countryside and everything that lived held its breath. The dogs' bark and donkeys' bay were silenced by the soft hand of the dark; the moisture dripping from the nude boughs stopped. I felt utterly dejected and alone, walking with time through an eerie silence in the shadow of the valley of death. So strong was my feeling of impending disaster that, moving as silently as the night about me, I lit the candles in the dual brass candelabras and stared into their golden centres until their halos of light blurred the edges of the room, casting my own image on the wall beside me. I watched myself climb into bed and turned my eyes to my clenched hands. I knew something was going to happen, just as I had known before Anthony's birth. Finally, I melted into sleep.

I could not dispel the foreboding of the previous evening and I said to mother, 'Something is going to happen.' She felt the same way. We were restless, waiting in anticipation. We knew each other too well to attempt to dispel such feelings with weak explanations.

We were expecting my elder brother Bob and his wife June, with niece Amanda, to call on their arrival at Heathrow Airport from Australia. Perhaps this explained our feeling? My younger brother, Tony, met them at Heathrow; they had arrived safely and we all exchanged Christmas greetings on the telephone. They couldn't come to stay with us for Christmas because of our isolation precautions to protect Anthony. They were off to Yorkshire to stay with June's family but they planned to come to Kent in mid-January, before they returned. They would stay at a guest cottage in the village overnight, just so we could see each other for a short while.

Events occurred to prevent that meeting ever taking place. How mother longed to be with her two sons, my elder brother Bob and my younger Tony (Anthony's namesake). It was not possible and we accepted it. One can get used to anything, even looking to our fourth Christmas alone.

At that time, David, our laboratory secretary, telephoned, extremely excited. Our donor register had been contacted for a compatibility test for an 11-year-old New Zealand boy, Leslie Dewhurst, due to arrive at Heathrow shortly and scheduled for a bone marrow transplant at Hammersmith Hospital in London. The doctors needed back-up cells for the transplant and we were elated that we could provide two supporting donors. The main donor for Leslie was his younger brother, Peter.

Eagerly we watched the arrival of Leslie, critically ill, drawn and barely able to walk, even with support. It was all on the national TV news. How well mother and I understood the mixture of feelings, fear and hope, of Mr and Mrs Dewhurst as they helped their son. Our Christmas prayers were for the success of Leslie's transplant, combined with our special prayers at Christmas for Anthony.

Alone we might have been that Christmas but not forgotten! A lovely young mother, Mrs Marilyn Newbury, with two beautiful daughters, wrote a moving and compassionate letter to the editor of the *Sun* newspaper in London. She asked that at Christmas everyone who cared should donate 50 pence towards our Appeal. Fifty pence. The price of that extra drink, a packet of balloons, a bauble for the Xmas tree. The *Sun* printed the letter and supported her appeal. Thousands of letters, donations and offers of help poured in from the length and breadth of Britain. Marilyn's thought for us led to the raising of more than £30,000 from *Sun* readers and helped ensure the completion of our laboratory renovations and a continuation of our work.

Here was another mother who cared … generating positive action. An individual who did prove that a small voice can, and will, be heard.

Brother Tony realised how desperately lonely mother must be feeling and drove down from the north to spend Christmas with us, after isolating himself for two days in his flat to check that he was free of influenza. It was so unexpected, so wonderful. His presence repainted Christmas. Mother busied herself preparing a superb lunch and I noted with a smile her happy singing as she clanged and clattered roasting dishes and pudding bowls. 'Rudolf', 'Jingle Bells' and Bing's 'White Christmas' seemed less hackneyed and doubly cheery as we sang with Anthony by the festive tree. Tony and I pulled Christmas crackers and clowned as we had in my student days. Anthony was delighted, cheering at each mini explosion until he rapidly detected the source and dismantled the box of crackers to collect the detonators.

Tony is an avid tea drinker and in Britain at the time was a particularly good and extremely amusing tea advertisement by PG Tips, using chimps dressed as humans and dubbed 'Tea, Mr Shifty'. Each morning, as his Uncle Tony appeared, Anthony would chorus, 'Cup-a-tea, Mr Shifty!' Anthony had just begun to be used to having Tony around when, after a week's stay, he had to leave. The next morning Anthony searched the cottage for him, then silently waited. The next day a closed look of resignation marked his little face. He'd been left again.

The first day of 1977 I awoke to Anthony's call but lay still for a while trying to accept a New Year. Yes, I would accept it but I would expect nothing from it.

Christmas and New Year were past. June and Bob were still in Yorkshire; Leslie Dewhurst was doing fine after his transplant in London. We were all flat out coping with the mail from the wonderful appeal by the *Sun* newspaper. Voluntary aides at the Westminster Hospital worked many hours sending out acknowledgements and leaflets explaining our work. Reporters from the *Sun* called frequently to record my reaction to the rapidly growing target of funds raised. I really couldn't express enough of my gratitude to Marilyn, the *Sun,* to all the thousands of caring people involved. The relief was like spring; the weight of my responsibility of supporting the running costs for our medical project at times drove me to panic and near despair. This was a reprieve and I could stop worrying for a while; we were solvent.

Late at night, after my Appeal work was completed, I lit the candles (this had become almost a ritual) and climbed into bed, sometimes fully clothed if I had worked to the limit. The flames soothed and painted the walls to soft orange, complementing the glowing coals in the black, carved hearth. The old books on the mantelshelves rippled in ridges of colour; each one well thumbed ... a novel, a book of poems, a classic. In that rare moment when

I stopped, between Anthony and the Appeal, I would reach out and remove the marker to read, perhaps, John Donne's 'Death Be Not Proud', or a section from my favourite play, 'Hamlet', D. H. Lawrence's 'Odour of Chrysanthemums', or Thomas Hardy's 'The Woodlanders'. Sliding between the sheets, the friendly smell of the printed pages close to my face, I would speak the words quietly aloud and slide sometimes back into the schoolroom when I shared such fruits of literature with my students. Usually I found the book the next morning dropped by the bedside as I fell asleep.

Saturday evening. Mother and I were clearing away in the kitchen, having settled Anthony for the night. I still had that strange feeling of anticipation, that something was going to happen.

'Mother ...' I said.

'Yes, I know,' she replied quickly. Our glances met; we had spoken thus before.

'How do you feel?' I asked.

'Overwhelmingly sad,' she said and sank to the floor on the hearth by the old kitchen stove. Usually, mother went off to bed or watched TV for a while as I headed to my table to work. I was poor company for her. Sadly, I never had any time to spare for her once Anthony was in bed. The Appeal work had to be done. But tonight I poured a drink for each of us and squatted opposite, my back against the fridge. Something was going to happen; we had both spoken our fears aloud and we both thought it was to be Anthony. I brought the day's unopened mail into the kitchen and poured a second drink. Instead of working alone I read the letters aloud to mother; I would answer them tomorrow. I remember one letter distinctly, from the mother of a boy of 13 living but a few villages away. He had died in tragic circumstances. She enclosed a donation to our work. Hardly able to continue reading, the pages blurred by mounting tears, I read of a son who always said flowers were wasted at funerals because the dead could not see their beauty. It was the opinion of a young boy and respected by his parents, family and friends, who made a donation to our Appeal instead of sending flowers to the funeral.

Mother and I were caught in a web of oppression drawing tighter and tighter. We sat talking quietly, slumped on the kitchen floor and had another drink, and another, trying to anaesthetise the growing feeling of horror.

Yet Sunday was Sunday as Sundays are, except that we both had a headache and the black shadow was still with us. That evening Anthony was in bed unusually early; I had tired him out with games of football down the hallway, bed-style trampoline, Pavlov's aeroplanes and ride-a-cock-horse. Mother looked unusually strained. I checked that Anthony was asleep, tucked him up and kissed his little fist through the cot bar, then turned on the TV and found a comedy play about to begin. I settled Mum on the settee and heard her chuckling while I made her night-time Milo. I handed her the steaming mug and returned to the kitchen to change Anthony's Milton solution and boil his drinking water. As the kettle came to the boil the telephone rang. Damn! I'd forgotten to put it on the low switch. I always did this as soon as Anthony was asleep.

I switched off the kettle at the instant mother screamed. My hands covered my mouth as I ran into the lounge. Mother was screaming, 'No, no, no!' and holding the phone away at arm's length. Just screaming at it.

'Mother ... Sshh,' I cried. 'Please, you'll wake Anthony ...'

'What is it, what? What's happened?'

I pulled the receiver from her, whispering, 'Hello, hello, who is it?'

'It's June.' My sister-in-law's voice from Yorkshire was like an automaton's, a level pitch steelily controlled. She had to repeat the dreadful words for me.

'Robert is dead ... he's been killed in a road accident.' Robert was their 16-year-old son, whose birthday had fallen just a few days before Christmas. My mother's only other grandson and my only nephew.

'How?' I asked.

'I don't know,' June replied. 'I'm waiting for the coroner's report … I must clear the line.' Click.

I quickly replaced the receiver and lifted mother back to the settee. She was muttering hysterically. 'I don't believe it … there's been a mistake.' Over and over again. She had snapped. She couldn't even see me.

'No, no,' she moaned. 'There's been a mistake. It must be a mistake.'

I shook out several sleeping tablets from my container and made her take them, talking to her all the time. 'Don't worry, Mum,' I said. 'I'll find out what's happened.' Then I steered her to bed. There was nothing I could do that evening. I knew June would phone if she wanted my help.

My nephew Robert had not wanted to go with his parents to visit England for Christmas. This beautiful boy, over six feet tall at the age of 16, with the rare combination of black hair and pale blue eyes, perhaps felt he was too old to go on holiday with his Mum and Dad. Instead of his holiday and air fare he'd asked for a motorbike as his Christmas gift. A lively, intelligent boy, he'd learned the highway code and passed his driving test at the first try. Crash helmets, I knew, were compulsory in South Australia, so what had happened? Early Monday morning I phoned Steve Foley, the London reporter for the Melbourne *Herald* newspaper group, covering the *Adelaide Advertiser*. Steve telexed to Australia for details. He called me back with the news.

A heat wave had hit Adelaide. Robert had been entertaining his friends at home, swimming in the pool followed by a barbecue. Still oppressively hot they had zoomed off into the Adelaide Hills on their bikes, where it would be cooler. It is a particularly exciting ride for youngsters on bikes … the roads snake around a chain of ponds – by day a scenic resort of blue lakes ringed by majestic pines, by night a death trap. Robert came off his bike as it skidded on gravel. No doubt embarrassed, as youngsters are at that age, he clambered on again to be dizzily thrown a second time. Leaving his bike, he was taken to his empty home on the pillion of a friend's machine and not to a hospital, even though they had to pass by the newly opened Modbury Hospital on their way. Robert had been wearing a crash helmet but had not fastened the strap. He had struck his temple in his fall.

At home, he climbed into bed. No one phoned a doctor. He was able to stagger out on Saturday morning but he, too, did not ring a doctor. Instead, he walked in what must have been a daze, the one-and-a-half miles to buy some Aspirin. Then he stumbled home again, took tablets for his aching head and died in his own bed, alone. It was a brain haemorrhage. His girlfriend found him the next day, Sunday. He had not turned up to collect her the previous night.

All this I learned from Steve Foley. Later the full tragedy was told. Although Robert was a mature and independent boy, June had asked friends Kath and Mick to check daily that all was well. Mick had called on the Saturday afternoon but seeing Robert's bike missing did not go into the house, assuming that all was well, when Robert was inside, dying. Mick phoned in the evening but Robert could not answer the phone.

I called Yorkshire and learned from June's mother that they left at dawn for Heathrow Airport to fly home. After her controlled call to me, June had collapsed.

Mother stumbled into the room, white and trembling, tears swelling in her eyes. I had to do something. All I knew was that June, Bob and Mandy were on their way to Heathrow. What a nightmare that drive must have been in winter from Yorkshire!

I was now terrified for their safety. Conditions were hazardous and with such tragic news and haste to return, I prayed for their well-being.

I looked at mother; she was sitting bolt upright, rigid, her face a deathly pallor, her mouth drawn back, her eyes staring. In stark contrast her hands were wringing out her grief and horror. I knew I had to snap her out of it. I phoned Heathrow and obtained the two flight times of the British Airways and Qantas flights to Australia. The next flight was at 6 p.m. The morning flight had departed. 'Mum, you must go to Heathrow,' I spoke, quietly and steadily. 'They need you … you can tell them what to do. Go and get yourself dressed and I'll call a taxi. You must go to Heathrow. Do you hear, mother? They need you.'

I called a taxi and told the driver to take mother to Ashford Station. They did all meet eventually, in the impersonal glare and bustle of Terminal Three at Heathrow. The tragic sight of her bewildered family jolted mother and she saw them on to their flight with the words: 'I will follow; I'll be with you.'

I played the day through with Anthony, fearing desperately now for mother's safety. Then I heard a car at the end of the driveway and familiar footsteps.

'There's my Nanna,' look said Anthony. Mother staggered in, her face lined with grief.

'I must leave,' she said. 'I have to be with them.' Anthony hugged his Nanna as I made her a strong cup of tea and listened to the little she could remember of the day's events. She could not recall her journey to and from Kent to Heathrow, only the meeting and her words: 'I will follow you.'

I was afraid now for Anthony and myself. How would we survive without Mother? Just the two of us, in winter? Yet I sensed she had to go or she would go insane. I had to think. I phoned my grandmother and asked her for the air fare; she contacted my brother Tony, who brought the money in cash to the cottage. I went up to London and booked Mum on the Qantas flight leaving on Wednesday for Australia.

We had been wrong. Our dark premonitions related not to Anthony, frail Anthony, clinging to life. It was a cruel twist of fate. It was beautiful, vibrant and healthy Robert. If Anthony, it would not have been unexpected. No less a loss but not unexpected. Of my mother's two grandsons, Robert died, not Anthony. The tragic irony is that Robert, like Anthony, suffered a brain haemorrhage in Adelaide, Australia, but no one was there to help him.

Wednesday morning. In a fever to be gone, mother was up before dawn. The silent night had buried Challock in feet of snow. I called a taxi but the roads were blocked; they were unable to conquer the hills to our village. In desperation, mother waded thigh deep in snow across the Lees to the village garage and the owner, bless him, drove her through the snow in his Land Rover to Charing, a railway station up the line. Thank God, the frequent day and night service to the south coast kept the lines open. Mother telephoned on her arrival at Heathrow. With relief I knew she would make the flight. Her flight into London with Anthony had been ghastly enough but how my family must have suffered with their thoughts on their return flights to Australia, sitting for hours unable to escape death waiting at the end of the journey.

In turn I called my brother Bob in Australia to tell him mother was on her way. I could barely recognise his voice, choked by his tragedy. Mother got there on Friday morning.

Before leaving our cottage she kissed Anthony goodbye. By evening he became restless and, drawing me to the window, called, 'Nanny, Nanny, Nanny.' He thought she was in the garden. It was dark, she should come inside. 'Nanny, Nanny,' he called. I knew he couldn't understand about Robert in Australia but he understood Linda and Auntie Dot, and so I tried to explain that Nanny had gone to see Auntie Dot. She would come back again.

He was reluctant to go to bed; he was tense, alert, listening. A car passed at the end of the driveway. 'There's my Nanny, look,' he cried.

'No, darling,' I explained. 'Nanny's gone away for a while but she'll come back again.'

Tony was able to stay the rest of the week and the weekend but had to return to university He had been a great comfort when Anthony had tottered down the hallway into Nanny's room, searching for her. He had found Tony instead and Tony made him laugh with his chimpanzee game of 'Tea, Mr Shifty', and helped me fill those anxious days by blowing balloons, cooking meals, carrying the heavy coal buckets and keeping fires blazing.

But Anthony was always looking and listening. At the arrival of the postman he eagerly ran to the door and his little face would close with disappointment when he didn't find his Nanna.

It was worse when Tony left. Anthony became more and more restless, calling and calling for his Nanna, sometimes to the point of hysteria, beckoning me again and again to the window and staring through at the wind and the rain, at the swaying boughs and through the rose arbour to Nanna's wood-cutting slab. He would prop his toes on the windowpanes to reach the latch which opened the small panes at the top and he called, 'Nanny, Nanny, Nanny,' to the unanswering garden, until with resignation, his face chilled from the draught, he turned away and sank into my lap.

I stroked his hair and sang and nursed him. Somehow I managed another week. The cottage alone needed constant attention. Two women had barely managed to keep it clean; for one it was too much. I usually cared for Anthony, his drugs and play, while mother cleaned, prepared meals and kept the fires going. The cottage had to be cleaned daily to remain as dust free as possible because of Anthony's allergies. The coal fires and the old stove generated sufficient ash and dust to occupy a housekeeper full time, so with mother gone I vacuumed, stoked fires, mopped kitchen floors, administered drugs, sterilised Anthony's crockery, fed him, played games, records and songs, cleaned out what appeared to be constantly blocked hearths and their mountains of ashes … on and on, interminable tasks.

Anthony awoke frequently during the night, calling for me, crying from his loss or another nightmare, and I sat on the floor and sang him to sleep with my head slumped against his cot bars. Sometimes I awoke stiffly at dawn, having fallen asleep like a rag doll against the cot.

The plop of the mail on the mat revealed the distinct blue of an aerogram from Australia. I picked it up and placed it in my apron pocket. It was Anthony's game to collect the mail and open envelopes for me; not that he could read, but he liked to examine the stamps and the varieties of shapes, weight and colour of the envelopes.

We were so alone. The mornings seemed an eternity, even bathing, feeding and just being with Anthony. He no longer wanted to play games. He was silent and clung to me desperately. I had to keep him beside me as I cleaned. He'd push the vacuum with me and kneel beside me while I shovelled out the piles of hot ash. He stood at the door watching me keenly, every second, as I hastily filled the coal buckets. He would not let me out of sight.

After having a restless night he fell asleep with me on my bed, his arms about my neck. Inch by inch I rolled until his arm gently dropped on to the covers.

It was afternoon before I could read the letter. Curled beside the fire I retrieved it, crinkled and blue, and slit the folds with my thumb nail.

Mother had arrived at Adelaide and was met at the airport by Ted. June and Bob were at their home, utterly distraught. Robert had been moved from the city morgue to a chapel of rest. They had not yet visited him. But together they gathered that Friday evening to witness Robert in death. After a journey of 12,000 miles, mother supported her son and daughter-in-law as they collapsed in their grief.

Finally, they were able to kiss their beautiful son goodbye, and mother her dead grandson. Each placed a rose in the coffin.

The words in the letter told more. Robert was unmarked; they had expected mutilation, signs of an accident, but there were none. He lay in his youth and beauty as if asleep. He was cremated on Saturday morning.

Robert was now an image in our minds. When we left Australia he was only 12 years old and I remember him calling outside the window where I sit now, writing this book: 'Nan, feel the stubble on my chin ... I'm shaving now.' He had laughed proudly, embarrassed by his broken voice faltering from boy to man.

I crumpled the letter in my palm and circled my knees with my arms and rocked to and fro, crying silently, not to wake my sleeping child.

Anthony became more and more disturbed. His Nanny had left him. She had been crying when she kissed him goodbye. Had he done something to hurt her; to make her angry with him so that she would leave him? Everybody left him. His Auntie Dot, his Tony, his Linda, even his Daddy, now his Nanna. With reproach and fear he stared at me. He must have been wondering if I would leave him as well.

I tried to control my grief. I tried to compensate for mother's loss but I was grieving inwardly for Robert and even more for the suffering of his family.

Children are incredibly perceptive. Surely Anthony could have sensed my grieving yet not have fully understood it? His Nanna was gone; I was grieving.

'Nanny will come back again,' I crooned to him over and over.

'Nanny, Nanny!' he awoke and called in the night.

Chapter 15

The lack of sleep, the constant physical drain of nursing Anthony, the domestic chores, and then the tantrums, were driving me towards a precipice. Life was like clinging to a rock-face with my bare fingernails, each one ripping off and leaving raw, bloody pulp. Anthony was distraught, tired and suffering. He frequently threw his Ribena drink at the wall, or on the carpet, or smashed his plate of toast, upturned his record player, threw anything he could find within reach, and bashed himself on walls, chairs, tables, doors, the bath rim. He even pinched his own face, bit himself ... anything to make the blood flow.

He had stopped calling for his Nanna and now he was punishing himself for driving her away or calling for her attention by self-inflicting wounds.

Streaks of sticky, messy Ribena were everywhere, mixed with spatters of Anthony's blood. I seemed to be eternally washing away blood stains. I understood, I shared his loss and I tried so hard to compensate. But one person, even a mother, cannot replace the world.

When calm, Anthony would patter down the hallway and I would find him curled up, eyes staring widely, on his Nanna's bed, waiting.

By the beginning of the third week Anthony was uncontrollable. He had walked up to the television – not switched on – and smashed his face on the screen and, streaming with blood, sent it toppling to the floor. I was terrified for his safety and yet angry at what he had done.

I picked him up, yelling at him, yelling at him on and on. I remember shaking him in my anger. Trembling, sobbing, I controlled myself and sang and calmed him and, nursing him as a baby, soothed him to sleep.

I couldn't stop my teeth chattering. The fires were now nearly out so I made a hot chocolate drink and realised it had been two days since I had eaten. I found some crackers and cheese and ate those, filled a hot-water bottle and climbed into bed.

In the in-between world of sleeping and consciousness I heard Anthony's call. Somehow I staggered to his room.

'I want a drink ... I want a drink!' he screamed. Barely able to see, despite the hall light always left on for him, I fumbled around in the kitchen and found his cup, made his Ribena and took it to him.

He grabbed the cup from me and flung it, deliberately, at the wall. I could see the scene like a slow-motion replay.

'No, Anthony, No!' I yelled. The stainless-steel cup clanged and the drink, like blood, spattered the wall. Just as slowly Anthony drew back his head and aimed his face at the rim of his cot. I tried to stop him but my hands moved in slow-motion also, and too late, they merely caught a spurt of blood.

All was red before my eyes ... the red of Anthony's brain haemorrhage spreading blooded rivulets. Screams! And red! A stranger's red ... those interminable drips from transfusions, on and on into Anthony, day after day, week after week, month after month, until he would burst, a blooded rose.

And Robert's death red, unseen red, river-flowing into the sea of death. And now, red everywhere, walls, floor, cot, clothes and Anthony's face. Screaming. A living stream of red. On and on. I grabbed him from his cot as he bashed his little fists into his face.

'Stop it!' I cried. 'Oh God, Anthony, stop it ... stop it ... stop it!'

I shook him and screamed at him as if to shake the very life out of him, until I crumpled on the floor.

'It should have been you, not Robert,' I shouted. 'My God, if you're going to die ... die! Damn it, DIE!'

The words were spoken. I crushed my face to his, my tears mingling with his blood, and kissed him over and over, and gathering him into my arms I stumbled down the hallway to nurse him by the fire.

I rocked him to and fro in the dim firelit room, my cheek pressed to his, and stroked the clotted fringe away from the now drooping eyelids. He was asleep and I backed on to the settee, still rocking and singing.

I held him close the rest of the night ... a night divided between fitful dozing and abrupt awakenings. I stared at the blood-caked face of my sleeping son, now appearing a horrifying black as the flood dried. I ran a fingertip over the flaked ridges and clotted nostrils, so that he had to breathe through his mouth. The quiet rhythm was still broken by intermittent sobs. I felt my own face, also tight and cracked with my son's blood and realised I had reached the end of a road.

Those words I had spoken aloud ... did I really wish Anthony dead? This little man I held in my arms all night, reluctant to be parted even to place him back in his cot?

It's been so long, I answered myself silently. I've been told so many times that he's going to die. I have waited for him to return from the operating theatre, sat by his bedside in hospital watching that constant stream of transfusions, listened for his death cry in the night, even held him in my arms believing him dead during terrifying seizures when he stopped breathing; and, when anaemic, holding my breath, I have bent my face to his to feel his breath on my cheek, so faint was the life within him.

And, worst of all, the haemorrhages, as my little boy and I battled a world through a sea of blood and I could see his life emptying, draining away.

I had lived his death so many times during the past five years. I had prepared myself for it. I had alternately steeled myself and cried until I felt wrung out, empty and useless as a discarded dried waterpouch in the desert.

Now I was in a desert. I had done all in my power for five years to keep Anthony alive. I had crossed the world with him and founded vital laboratories. I would even die for him. Yet, incredulously, I had this night wished him dead and almost killed him. And I would always have to return to that desert of my guilt, whether Anthony lived or died.

The words had been spoken. The thought, not carried through to action, was still the same.

I called my doctor and he arrived to find us locked together in blood. I gently swabbed Anthony's face and changed his stained clothes, not caring about my matted hair and the dishevelled appearance. The doctor asked where mother was. His, 'Oh, no,' as he sadly stroked Anthony's head was summary enough.

'I can't cope any more,' I said. 'I nearly killed Anthony last night.' He stared at me intensely. 'You must realise that ordinary mothers with ordinary children sometimes feel as you do,' he said. 'I am surprised you have exercised so much control for so long.'

'But how could I say or feel such a thing?' I asked. 'Believe me, my dear,' he went on, 'there is no need to recriminate yourself – it's really more common than you think.'

Common! God, I thought, he really doesn't understand. I stared hopelessly about me. The fires all needed stoking, the ashes emptying, and Anthony's cot was wet and bloodstained. Sticky Ribena coated the walls and floors. It would take me most of the day to clean Anthony's room alone. If I didn't disinfect it scrupulously, the spiders and ants were attracted to the dripulets of sugary blackcurrant juice. I closed my eyes and visualised the scrubbing away at bloodstains and a bath full of blood-soaked baby clothes and linen. The washing machine was outside and I had to do the washing in the bath or boiler. In the winter those voracious fires needed constant stoking just to keep the place warm. It was as if they were burning away our lives.

'Doctor, I just can't go on,' I cried.

'You must,' he replied. 'Anthony needs you.' He was right, of course. How could I fail Anthony now with the loss of his Nanna, knowing also her knife-edge mental condition when she left? How could she cope with the betrayal of her only grandson, sick and frail as he may be? I had to keep Anthony alive for his sake and hers.

'But you must have help,' the doctor continued. 'Do you have any friends who can come and stay with you?' I thought, No, no, I do not. Any friends had moved along with life over the past five years. Anthony and I are here, left behind alone. The only other person who could possibly understand was 12,000 miles away, mourning her dead grandson and calming her children. My only friend since college days, who had never lost contact with me, was Freida, who was in mid-term teaching and also had two young daughters to look after on her own. She would have come but it was not possible. My relatives, including Linda, were far in the north of Yorkshire, all ill with influenza.

We were alone, terribly alone. And I was afraid to be left alone. I remembered the agency nurses used in London.

'A nurse,' I burst out to the GP. 'Do we have a nursing agency locally? I must have a resident nurse.'

'You do realise they are a costly private expense and not covered by the National Health Service?' he replied. I didn't care. 'Please call the agency,' I said. That evening June, a Devonshire lass – young, pretty and cheery – arrived. I was hoping she would be informal and adaptable and, thank God, she was. Anthony has never allowed anyone to bathe, feed or treat him but me, with the exception of his periods in hospital. His Nanna could sing and nurse him but only his mother was allowed to touch him. June settled in and cleaned up the mess, washed the clothes, emptied the ashes, filled the coal buckets and cooked atrocious meals. But she was terrific and a breath of normality. Anthony loved her.

Once order was restored we played for hours with his tipper truck and a bag of dried peas, spilling them all over the lounge floor. While I ran Anthony through them chuckling as he spun them with his toes, June collected the piles over and over again.

June slept in mother's room – and like a log. Being so used to listening for Anthony I would wake first, stoke the fires, make June a cup of tea in bed and then collect Anthony, who would head for June's room to drag his new playmate out of bed. June was a tremendous help. I am truly grateful that she did not object to being the domestic while I continued as nurse.

Anthony had stopped calling for his Nanna and turned for attention to June. But, during our play, he would stop, a haunted look on his face, and drift to the window to squash his face to the glass and stare into the grey of the day or the black of the night. The weeks stretched away interminably. I now had to be Anthony's world. We would be listening to music, dancing or playing a game, apparently happy; then, like a trigger shot, a memory would blast him and his laughter dissolved into hysterical head-banging, splattering blood everywhere. The only solution was to place him in his cot, which I had now padded, where he could do himself least harm, half-crying, half-cursing, I waited for the calm while cleaning up the mess.

I knew Anthony was now walking a dangerous tightrope. He could not continue his sad life for much longer. It was as cruel and effective as solitary confinement. An innocent, he had served a five-year prison sentence. We had existed on hope, the three of us, keeping one step ahead of Anthony and his predicted death. Now death had dealt a below the belt blow and we were all floundering beneath its force. For once I admitted to myself that I was nearing the end of the line.

The next letter from mother told of their grief. They blamed themselves for Robert's death, for leaving him. If they had not been away perhaps he would have been saved. At least everything possible would have been done.

Mother felt she could not leave them yet; their heartache was too great. She said she was afraid my brother Bob would take his own life. At night she would listen to him sobbing on the bed where his only son died.

I read and re-read the letter and cried alone in my bed. I had several times expected Anthony's death and remembered the agony of the imagined loss. Now I was living with their suffering across the world and I felt as if the world was weeping. I wept for them, for my lost nephew, my son, and all humanity, lost in the depth of their suffering.

In the third letter, mother said she wanted to return but felt she was needed more in Australia.

In those first weeks alone I had kept from her Anthony's alternate periods of depression and aggression. I pretended that I was managing with June's help but as the weeks passed I could now see myself plummeting down a rock-face of defeat. For 18 hours a day Anthony never left me.

Even with June's help the biting and banging would rise to the surface and erupt in agonising red hysteria.

After two months I asked mother to come back. My brother Bob was to be admitted to hospital; he did not care if he lived or died. He would be carefully watched.

* * *

Mother walked in looking tired from the long journey. Anthony ran away from her and hid his face in the hollow of my shoulder. She had left him and two months is a lifetime to a child, especially Anthony. She had rejected him, as he saw it, and now he rejected her.

June overlapped the return by a week until, gradually, Anthony accepted his Nanna back again but she was not the Nanna who had left. How could she be after such an experience? Anthony, too young to comprehend, but able to sense a change, tried to draw the previous love and attention but mother was drowning in the loss of her other grandson. Anthony would amble down to her room and find her sobbing on her bed or she would suddenly collapse in tears and Anthony would approach her and place his head on hers, as if to say he was sorry, a puzzled expression on his face, as if he was the cause of her grief; or perhaps he understood more than we imagined.

His disturbed behaviour and demands for attention were now continuous, his self-aggression horrifying. He smashed his fists into his face, bit his arms and legs until he was bleeding and purple-black bruised. I couldn't even shower; he would draw my attention in some way. My long, shoulder-length hair became matted and unmanageable. I called the village home hairdresser and she came and cut it all off, down to an inch. I stared at my thin face, the shadows and lines, my cropped head and I couldn't recognise me. I looked like a prison inmate but I lifted my head and I glared back at my image. I didn't care, I would not be beaten. It was not what I looked like that counted.

The days passed in wiping the blooded cot, walls and floors and I became more and more angry with mother for not controlling her grief, if only for Anthony's sake. I cried occasionally, when rock-bottom low and lonely, but with my head under the pillow. Before my nephew Robert's tragedy, when I had worked late hours for the Appeal, mother did what we called the dawn shift, leaving me in bed until the morning tea was made. Now she could not stir. I had to work into the small hours and with only four to six hours sleep, collect Anthony, change him, stoke the fires and try to fix the mask of normality for the day. But it slipped awry. My poor little son's confusion was pitiful to witness as he tried to drag his Nanna out of bed, from the drugged sleep dulling her cruel memories.

The demands for the Appeal were more pressing yet I feared to leave Anthony and mother alone. As a consequence, when it was essential to travel to London for a meeting of the committee of the Anthony Nolan Trust I would fit in several press interviews, visit personalities in London theatres, broadcast on Radio London and do a final interview for the six o'clock television news. It was a week's work in one day. I would feed Anthony before I left and administer his drugs. I knew he would then play for a while and have an afternoon nap, tired because of his nightmare-disturbed sleep. At night, I would be back to bathe, feed, nurse and play with him until he finally gave in to go to his room. This was signalled by his, 'On my mark, Mummy.' I would reply, 'Right, ready, steady, go!' and he would gallop through the lounge and down the long hallway into his Nanna's room and kiss her goodnight as she lay in the darkness to dim her memories.

Frequent power cuts often extinguished Anthony's night light, causing him to awaken in the cold and darkness. I began to leave a candle burning in his room and the soft light soothed him. Each evening I lit the taper in a heavy old brass candlestick, originally found damaged, corroded and discarded in the tower of a church my younger brother used as a studio. Mother had scraped and polished for weeks to restore it.

Now I stared at the silhouette of its serrated rim, stretching across the shiny floor, and its gently changing shaded shape at the candle's whim, which duplicated the cot bars on the bedroom wall and across Anthony's sleeping face, like an ominous birthmark. I stroked his ruffled hair and tiptoed out.

Then there would be the difficult nights. 'I want a drink,' he would say and, splat, it would stain the wall. 'Close the curtains, open the curtains, light on, light off,' followed by brutal poundings on the eighteen-inch padded foam. I knew his dilemma and I over-compensated for it by unending patience, tolerance and care. I thought I was being understanding but, really, he was crying out for help, for guidelines. He needed a behaviour parallel not a desert of tolerance.

After one vital committee meeting in London, I returned to rural Kent to find the cottage in total darkness. My heart thumping, I entered the kitchen to find mother slumped on the floor, crying and singing, on and on, rocking Anthony. I spoke to her but she could not hear me. She was with the dead. I was angry with poor mother. Feel it but for God's sake don't show it, I wanted to scream. I gathered Anthony into my arms, flicked on the lights and jollied him to reaction. I filled a hot-water bottle, made a hot drink then steered mother to bed.

I bathed and fed Anthony, played our number and letter games and his favourite records and, finally, stroked him to sleep. I knew I could not leave mother alone again. I stared at the pile of unopened mail, pushed it aside and, unwashed, crawled into bed.

It was to be the night of the storm. I awoke to a lightning flash, fierce as a flicked razor across my eyes. I soothed Anthony, who clung to me, cowering at each brilliant flash and the ensuing crack and roll of thunder. By now, mother – also terrified by storms – was frantically raking embers and soon had the two lounge and dining room fires blazing. I have never witnessed such a magnificent storm. It passed directly over Challock and the ground reverberated with the force of the thunderclaps, while rain lashed and rattled the windows.

I thought, let the heavens fall, come Armageddon, we welcome it. I said to mother, sitting quietly, 'It's like the end of the world.'

'And I am ready,' she replied.

* * *

I don't know when I first noticed the hair on my shoulders and on my pillow each morning. It's your imagination, I spoke to my image in the bathroom mirror. Combing gently, I held the crop of hair in my hands. It was true. My hair was falling out. I'd always had such a mane of hair and, with irony, recollected my cursing that it was so thick and unmanageable. Now it was thin and lifeless and I stared at the dead strands in my palm. Strangely, I didn't care. I didn't care a damn. What does anything matter anymore, I thought? Then, stop thinking like that, pull yourself together. Mother and Anthony desperately need help.

'Mother, you must see a doctor,' I said next morning. I didn't mention my hair. Mother was fortunate in having a wonderful lady doctor who listened and cared and carefully prescribed anti-depressants.

I wrote to Anthony's paediatrician in my quarterly report to London and stated that he was seriously disturbed. No action was taken. I tried to compensate with my love, but it was second best, parrying with my conflicting emotions of grief for my nephew, my family in Australia, mother suffering and my concern for her loss and conflict. I tried harder and harder, but I couldn't help mother. She went about in a daze. The drugs sedated her and she barely managed to cope with each day as it came. It was absolute hell. She was living with her dead grandson. And I wanted to scream, 'But your only other grandson is alive and needs you; you must think of him, you must.'

Watching Anthony suffering, and her despair, for the first time I contemplated suicide for the three of us. It was the only way we could escape and be together, so inextricably were our lives intertwined. Later, when she improved a little, on one of our rare peaceful evenings, mother, aghast, admitted that she had been thinking the same.

My hair continued to fall out until I was bald on the front and on my crown. Each time I washed my hair I watched more and more disappear until I stopped looking in the mirror. It was happening, that was all.

Chapter 16

In spring I was most fortunate to find a woman in the village to come in and help five days a week. Tiny, plump and jolly, Berta's smiling face appeared through the door with a 'Hullo cocker,' for Anthony and, rolling up her sleeves, she set about with force, mopping, sweeping and vacuuming. Generally, Anthony was beside her. He especially liked wiping the small windowpanes, copying Berta, or she would guide him along with the vacuum. She was kind, patient, sympathetic and a tremendous help to Mum and Anthony simply by her bubbly personality.

Gradually mother began to improve and I was able to continue my work for the Appeal with interviews by telephone or paperwork late at night. I was asked to write a television script for BBC 2, 'The Light of Experience'. It was an appropriate theme. I had to write about how my life had changed since Anthony's birth, and my values and attitude towards life.

The 5,000-word script highlighted just how much my life had changed. My pride and independence were gone. But were they such a loss? The resilience of youth was gone. I had always felt I could conquer the world. Whatever I wanted I could achieve; I was invulnerable. This was my arrogance. Now I realised ambition was empty fruit, that confidence was a facade which could crack. I was vulnerable and the one thing I now desired more than the world was my son's life – and I couldn't give it to him. He had grown within me for nine months and during those months I had, at times, allowed myself to dream, to plan what he would look like, the colour of his hair, his eyes, how he would look at me, how I would care for him. I'd even imagined his first day at school, a sturdy boy, as I proudly waved goodbye. I had imagined my returning to teaching, which I enjoyed so much, and enjoying the full life that is so taken for granted ... a busy teacher, a mum and wife, my days crammed as they had been with interest, variety, vitality and zest for life.

I was describing a person I no longer recognised as I wrote the script and wondered how I had come to the end of the road. I had always loved life to the full, but I now wished to squash it like a rotten fruit, toss it out of the window, even murder my son. Of course, I couldn't put this in the script. It wasn't appropriate and possibly wouldn't have been believed, anyhow.

Always pictured as the brave, battling super-mum it was impossible to project the part of me I had to hide – the lonely, the almost-defeated and the desperate. I wouldn't be pitied; I would die first.

It was at this time of abject despair that I received a letter – the second – from Kathy, who headed a prayer group in Australia. It contained a pressed daisy because they had heard it was Anthony's favourite flower. The first one I had read, as usual, late at night. It was typed in capital letters, words missing and askew. I had read and re-read it. She said that life can be like a desert, empty, meaningless but it is only in a desert, metaphorically, that we can find our true selves, stripped of the world man has constructed. We must then examine the world within. I remember the letter because at the time of reading it, I felt exactly as she described. I was sitting in that desert, picking myself to pieces like a carrion crow. I laughed to myself at the trivia that had once troubled me: an untidy house, washing to be done, piles of examination papers to be marked, a personality clash at work, the resulting arguments, the irritant of individual mannerisms and so on. When picked clean of my conditioning the basics were so simple. Life, health and truth.

The second letter contained the words, 'It is so easy to kill a child.' How had Kathy known what I was thinking? The thought was hard enough to bear, but the printed words witnessed my horror and guilt. I had received hundreds of letters during my years of isolation from religions all over the world. I had replied with thanks and asked them to pray for Anthony. I prayed for Anthony every night and for all sick children everywhere, but I now see that, in all honesty, I thought myself too unworthy for God to hear and answer my prayers. Why should He when I alternately cursed him and then begged for Anthony's life? The truth is that I didn't understand. In many ways I still don't.

What I did understand now is that we have a choice between good and evil, that we would be automatons if we all behaved the same as if we had no free will. God had not created the evil that had resulted in Anthony's illness. Man had. God had given talents and brilliant men had found a cure for Anthony's illness. God was not now preventing his treatment. Man was. Gradually I was beginning to understand that as a parent we can try to guide, to help, our children but they must choose the path they wish to take. So it is with God's children. I read the ensuing letters from Kathy and her little group, named the 'Daisy Group,' but I still believed myself unworthy. I was only a half-believer, anyway.

My so-called faith moved like the tide touching the shores and receding. Always the question would arise: 'If God wanted me to do his work and serve a purpose by helping suffering children, why did it have to be through the suffering of my son?' I had wanted to end his suffering by killing him and then myself. I would not wish to live without him. I had blatantly advocated euthanasia in my student days – my days of health, light, love and laughter – the apparently superior destroying the inferior. I believed that quality of life was paramount. My own words echoed and mocked me. Now, where is your quality of life? What is important, purely and simply, is LIFE. I still wanted life for my son.

* * *

In June, 1977, I began trying to obtain home tuition for Anthony. A teacher was finally allocated for two hours a week. It was all that could be arranged. Invariably, Anthony was asleep when she arrived at midday. I had settled him in his cot one day as she arrived. I had tried to keep him awake. I asked if she could try to change the schedule to see him in the mornings after seven or by one p.m., his nap time. She was a sweet lady with a large family of her own but said the Department made the rules. Really, I wasn't listening anymore. This department, that department, yet Anthony appeared to be nobody's responsibility. A forgotten one, a child who, by rights, shouldn't be alive at all. I was pleading for help for him and no one was able to help.

If what I had seen as I stroked his head as he fell asleep was a reality any help was now too late. There were several pink, shiny patches beneath his luxuriant hair. As the teacher left I called our doctor. Before Anthony awoke I spoke with him in the kitchen. He was concerned about my weight loss, asked if we ate regular meals and arranged for me to see a specialist about my hair. I nodded without commitment and led him to Anthony's room. As he rolled sleepily, the doctor gently lifted his thick strands of hair and then confirmed my fears. Anthony had been off his steroid drugs for more than three months. I had almost dismissed my fears of any side effects. His puffy, steroid face had returned to the tiny face so little changed from the day of his birth. His thin legs had filled out to complement his broad shoulders so that he appeared a sturdy toddler, his size belying his age. He looked like a bonny three-year-old.

My first thought was that I had a scalp infection which I had passed on to Anthony. 'No,' said the doctor. 'Alopecia is not contagious; your hair loss is due to stress and fatigue. We must observe Anthony and hope that his loss is only minor.' But Anthony's hair continued to fall out rapidly. When I held him close, his head on my breast, I gazed with concealed horror at the tangled mass of dark hairs left on my blouse. The bald patches grew larger and larger, thinning the thick, beautiful hair, leaving it lank and lustreless. Our doctor had contacted the Children's Hospital in London, but I was reluctant to submit Anthony to more distress.

The decision was, strangely, made for me. Two potential donors were found for Anthony, one through our donor session in Sussex, the other a Dutchman from our European connections. Both were good matches. The transplant team in London expressed the opinion that, due to Anthony's deterioration, and the necessity to take blood from him for the final compatibility tests, it would be advisable to admit him to hospital, await the results and, at the same time, examine and observe him.

Four years had passed since I had first climbed those steps into the Westminster Children's Hospital, clutching Anthony with such heartache. Now we were here again.

The examinations and ghastly bleeding sessions completed, Anthony was not in a pre-transplant environment. Everything he needed was in the small room. Food and linen were sterilised. Before entry the nurse opened one container and, without touching it, I took the inner container, with anything inside from a towel to a slice of bread or a mini honeypot. Outside the cubicle were containers of sterilising solution so that stainless steel equipment and bottles could be submerged the required time. Before they entered the room, staff and visitors had to be covered head to foot in hair-caps, masks, ankle-length gowns, plastic gloves and plastic shoe covers. All that was left visible were the eyes. Pre-warned, the cot had been padded with pillows and had to be changed again and again as Anthony battered his fears on the bars.

His hair now fell out in handfuls. Stroking his head, my hand fell away with a lump of hair. The floor was like a barber's shop until, and the end of a week, apart from a wisp here and there, Anthony was completely, tragically bald. I could now see quite clearly, like a map of the past, the scars circling his head from his brain surgery; neat, white lines as a witness of his suffering.

I had talked with Anthony's new paediatrician on admission. I stressed that Anthony was seriously disturbed. Arrangements were made to see the Child and Family Psychiatry Department. Unfortunately, this kind, understanding paediatrician was now due for summer leave. I was introduced to his representative. I had been able to talk with the senior paediatrician and I respect the way he spoke frankly with me about Anthony. I felt that his junior regarded me as just another fussy mother.

The first tests on the Sussex man rejected. They had been unable to trace the Dutchman. He was a travelling salesman. We had to wait for a second bleeding. I saw the psychiatrist and told her Anthony's case history, mother's tragedy, our family break-up and, explicitly, about both my screaming at Anthony to die and my fear of killing him – killing all of us. I desperately wanted help.

It was not easy to make such frank admissions. I was hoping to God the psychiatric treatment would now begin, to help my little boy. I could see by her look she thought I was dramatising, but she agreed Anthony needed help. I asked her if someone could see Anthony for a little while each day, to observe him and to guide me to the best way of helping him.

'But we have no one available,' she said. 'Our department is understaffed and overworked. The best I can do is to see him myself and assess him.' Assess him, I thought. I know what he is! He is physically and developmentally a three-year-old with a five-year-old inside, screaming to be let out, and he is extremely disturbed and soon, very soon, he is going into a corner to give up the fight, curl up and wish to die. With what yardstick could Anthony be assessed against the normal five-year-old? What other child had been in solitary confinement for most of his life? It wasn't assessment I needed: it was positive and speedy help.

I was again pleading for help for Anthony; he was crumbling before me. Wild-eyed, bald, bleeding, battered and ulcerated, he was like a little old man. Tests showed that he had bone structure deficiency, little surprise after years of drugs and severely restricted diet. With his paediatrician on leave and no psychiatrist to help him, and the need to chase around Europe a Dutchman who could save his life, the future looked grim. It was decided that I might be too strong an influence on Anthony and his not eating a way of punishing me for allowing him to suffer so since birth. I had to admit that this theory had crossed my mind more than once. But why had he had such a voracious appetite as a toddler before his journey to London?

Mother was to stay at the hospital with Anthony, but I had to leave him completely for a week. His diet then was toast, Bovril and Ribena.

I returned alone to the empty cottage. I wasn't overjoyed at having the place to myself or the time to do as I wished. I didn't know how to handle time without Anthony. Without my son I did not exist. But the experiment had to be tried. I spent the days doing jobs that had been left unattended. I repainted timbers ravaged by two long winters, cleared the mail, played scrabble, and listened to my favourite piano music. In the evenings I stared at the world on television, the world with which I was now out of step. Those days alone also gave me time to think.

Chapter 17

My day was spent impatiently waiting for the evening phone call from mother. For seven days Anthony did not eat a scrap of food. The staff tried everything from coaxing to force-feeding. I had heard enough. I returned to London. 'Oh, God, how much am I expected to bear? What is your will? Why, why?' I screamed again in my head as I stared through the glass into the isolation cubicle at my five-year-old, curled foetal position, grey, bald, emaciated and brutally bruised. My images flashed like the closing of an eyelid – that day long ago when I ran from the sight of my baby a few days old, similarly curled in an incubator.

I didn't don the gown and mask to see him. I had changed my clothes in the mothers' unit. He had to see *ME,* not just as two eyes and a gowned figure. This time I did not want to run away. I flicked on the shoe covers and opened the door.

'Anthony, my Anthony, baby, Mummy is here, Mummy is back again,' I told him. He turned his head as I approached and I lowered the cot bars and lifted him out, cradling his tiny form like a baby.

'I'll give you a daisy a day,' I sang. Our eyes met; he was very weak. I ordered sterilised milk, Weetabix and honey and I stayed with him late into the night until he took the first spoonful, then a little more and a little more. Finally I sang him to sleep.

At seven the next morning, I ran down from the mothers' unit and began again. He ate a full Weetabix and a third of a pint of milk with honey. I nursed him all morning and never left him. He sensed that I was not only back with him physically but that my will had gathered strength. Our struggle to survive was on again.

Mother was wonderful. Spending such a week with Anthony, witnessing him sink day by day, had snapped her out of her grief. No, she was not going to lose her only other grandson without a fight either. We all sensed it, we three. We were a team again. We would not give in.

The Dutchman was found and the test tube simulation began. Anthony ate Weetabix, milk and honey, nothing else, but lots of it and he gained weight and filled out again. The sisters and nurses were wonderful and we all eagerly awaited the results of the tests.

Two other patients were in hospital at this time, an 18-month-old boy and a 14-year-old Indian girl. Both children, critically ill, were being sustained in sterile plastic bubbles as neither of them had a donor. In the mothers' unit I eagerly sought news of the children, especially the young girl. Her mother, petite and beautiful in her sari, told me the next day that as a last chance the doctors were going to use her as the donor, so critical was her daughter's condition. Even in their sadness they eagerly asked about my work. Their daughter was in the same category as Anthony, potentially curable but for lack of a donor. Our common bond was our love for our children. Race and religion were no barrier. We shared the evening.

The next day their daughter died. Oh God, how many more? Now the isolation bubble was empty. Was it destined to be so for Anthony?

During this waiting period of six days for the results, mother said she could not face the prospect of another winter's isolation. Not only was she helping her grandson but she was burdened with the worry of her son. He was still unwell and had not returned to work. My sister-in-law was supporting the family. I knew that mother wanted to return to be with them. I knew Anthony also could not survive another winter's isolation, so I vowed that if these tests rejected we would try to return to Australia to join my brother and his family and avoid another winter alone.

The tests on the Dutchman proved unsuitable so I contacted my Australian friend, Steve Foley of the Melbourne *Herald* group in London, and told him how much we desperately wanted to return to Adelaide. The Adelaide *Advertiser* had covered Anthony's story since the spring of 1973. They had taken the first Press photo of him and written the first story. They did not fail us. The *Advertiser* and the 'Willesee at Seven' television show sponsored us back to Australia.

Frenzied preparations ensued at my brother's farm near Gawler, 25 miles north of Adelaide. My two brothers and June worked from dawn to dusk to block in the double carport to make a unit for me and Anthony. Mother packed and sent essentials ahead. I had to write to Anthony's former paediatrician and arrange for his medical case notes to be forwarded. I planned the flight and our needs to the last detail, gave interviews to Steve about our preparations, and organised the Appeal so it could be kept running in my absence.

At four o'clock on the morning of our departure Steve arrived at the cottage with the hire car and, with the driver, loaded our mountain of boxes and suitcases and the colossal travel bag containing everything from Anthony's gallon of sterile water to pre-cooked toast, favourite toys and even his potty. We set off in the now chill, misty October morning for Heathrow. Anthony is a terrific traveller and watched eagerly the headlights approaching and receding in the dark and then the more numerous lights as we approached the city and dawn. He didn't fall asleep. He somehow knew he wasn't going back to hospital. He sensed our anticipation. We were like birds released from their tiny cage and soon we were to soar into the morning sky. I had a feeling we had forgotten something and a few miles from Heathrow I realised it was Anthony's stainless-steel cup. He would only drink out of this one special cup. The hire car driver had to pass the Royal Marsden Hospital so we tried there. They had nothing similar. He then had an idea. As he lived close by he called at his home. He had a large collection of pewter beer tankards and, from a selection, I chose one I thought may suit our needs. All was prepared at Heathrow. Camera crews in full force had set up in the conference room but Anthony was now edgy, darting startled looks about him. He tugged at the steering wheel; he wanted to keep moving. 'Move, Mummy, move,' he said. While he was moving, he was out of his prison. To stop meant a return to it. I had to decline the conference room firmly and the cameras were brought to the car. We were filmed while seated. Then, with police escort, we were taken to the medical unit and, by ambulance car, direct to the plane now due for take-off on the runway. Placed on a special lift, we rose up to meet the plane, its huge rounded shiny side like the belly of a whale.

This was the spot the press photographers had chosen for their departing shots. We walked directly into the first-class section without having to climb a step, so superb were the arrangements for Anthony's journey. We moved to our seat in the nose of the 747. The engines were revving for take-off, then ceased. We were delayed.

Passengers noted with interest our dramatic entrance and now, between speedy glances and averted eyes, their faces reflected mixed reactions. Pity, horror, revulsion, curiosity and indifference. My head ached, we had been up since four and it was now 10 a.m.

An unusually bright sun seared the sky and the aircraft became warmer and warmer. Anthony began to fidget; he wore only a singlet and a velour shirt to his hips. No pants, no shoes. He was bald and marked cruelly with eczema. He pulled off his shirt and then his singlet. Innocent and overheated, he had removed his clothes and stood, scarred, for all to see. For a moment I felt a blush of embarrassment. What would the passengers think? Eczema is such an unsightly complaint. Come now, I told myself. You have to travel 12,000 miles to keep this little fellow alive. It doesn't matter what people think. You have to cross the world and hope you have made the right decision. If you have made the wrong one then you have killed your son, just as surely as if you had shot off his head.

By tempting him with distilled ice drinks I had prepared for the journey, I managed to keep Anthony in our space in the nose of the aircraft. Despite his tragic appearance, we, fellow passengers and crew, had a laugh at our little fellow, quaffing his drink out of a beer mug. He laughed on take-off at the thrust and pull-back of the powerful engines and, once in motion, again sat happily on my lap and watched the coastline of England recede and clouds brush past.

At a higher altitude the cabin cooled and Anthony put back his singlet and shirt. By now the stewards had been tactfully pumped and once the passengers realised it was Anthony, or that the little boy up front had something similar to leukaemia, and it was not infectious, everyone relaxed and I was able to allow Anthony to leave our comer. He fearlessly explored each new face and quickly found the spiral staircase to Captain Cook's cabin. I do not exaggerate when I write that the first leg of the journey of about eight hours from London to Bombay we ascended and descended that spiral staircase, toured the cabin, swivelled the seats and toured the cabin below. The only problem during the flight were the two movies. Anthony wanted his porthole curtain open and the light affected the screen. So I did another two hours up and down the magic staircase. During the second film he wanted to sleep and the flickering screen disturbed him but we managed to sing him to sleep.

Taxiing into Perth Terminal I could see clearly the Press gathered in force. I had to carefully descend the staircase to the tarmac, holding Anthony my precious cargo. My legs felt as if they were walking several steps ahead and the bright sunlight blinded me. I clutched the rail firmly with one hand and Anthony more firmly with the other. We were ushered without ceremony into the conference room. Questions were fired at me from all angles, cameras whirred and flash bulbs burst. I answered as best I could and, for once, found myself stuttering. I handed Anthony to Mum, out of the heat of the camera lights, but he began to struggle and call for me, and mother looked irritated so I called a halt.

A doctor then arrived to examine Anthony. We would not know for at least 48 hours if he had contracted an infection. The doctor was not needed. Our guide steered us through the terminal for the final stage of our journey from Perth to Adelaide. The officials were kind and helpful but had not, as in London, gauged our transference with such care. As a result I had to walk through the crowded terminal cradling my exhausted son asleep in my arms. Mothers with children pulled away as if Anthony were a leper. Perhaps they just thought he was dead. Perth was very hot for October and I had to walk a kilometre to the aircraft standing blurred and shimmering in the heat haze. On the tarmac we were allowed to board before the other passengers and were allocated the front row again in the nose of the plane. I somehow staggered up the steps and collapsed, panting, in my seat. Anthony was a tiny five-and-a-half-year-old weighing only 16 kilos but, after such a journey from London, it took every scrap of reserve to board the plane.

Chapter 18

Mother said: 'I can see it.' Turning my head, as the plane dipped, still over the sea, Adelaide was clearly visible. We have made it, I whispered inwardly. The pocket-handkerchief gardens, the dolls' houses and the matchbox cars all revolved until we thumped on the runway. I could see so clearly the Creek kids, our neighbours' children, who had remembered Anthony all the time we were away, holding their hand-painted sign, 'Welcome Home Anthony!' I waved to my neighbours, well-wishers and friends at the airport. Our car left the runway and parked at the front of the terminal. My neighbours, and the babies I remember now grown to young boys and girls, presented their beautiful bouquets of flowers. I looked at the tired little fellow on my lap and at his tall, bouncing, healthy contemporaries and realised the difference. But it was so good, so very good, to see them all after so long.

Two people I did not see who awaited our arrival at the terminal were Anthony's father, hidden from view, and dear Kathy, who had travelled in all the way from Berri with a cluster of daisies for our welcome from her prayer group. To learn of her gesture afterwards was to appreciate its significance.

The car headed for Willaston, near Gawler. Anthony was still and happy again in motion. Now I felt a stranger, thrust from rural Kent back to Australia, the Australia I loved. Dave, from the *Advertiser,* asked Anthony how he felt. He tossed back, 'Sick as a dog,' and, in true Australian fashion, said no more. We turned off the bitumen and on to the dirt road to my brother's farm. The sun was directly in our eyes, silhouetting the gnarled gums, a crazy· black fretwork against its burnt orange backdrop. We stopped, followed by folds of bulldust as the dogs came charging out, baying and snapping at the cars, until chained by my brother. I noted the dull eyes and slower step. Dear Bob, never much one for words. He greeted us and said, 'I'll put the kettle on.

The double carport was now a self-contained unit with a large lounge, sleeping area and a kitchenette. The long spacious back verandah had been fly-screened to provide a fresh-air, insect-free play area for Anthony. They had done a marvellous job.

June sat up most of that night finishing the lovely handmade raffia lamp shades for our room, but still my heart sank as the cars left. As the sun sank behind the now-unfamiliar gum trees I instantly realised we had simply changed our location from isolation in Kent, England, to Willaston, South Australia. At least we are not alone, I said to myself. At least we have the summer to look forward to, not another bitter winter. Mother is back where she has yearned to be and, I thought, if Anthony is meant to die it is appropriate that he dies in the place of his birth.

My family had spent all making a home for us. They had been helped by Solomons, who provided vinyl floor covering, Malley's, who gave a fridge and a local lady who had paid for the glass for the windows.

The bulk of the expense for the conversion, on top of all their problems, the family had borne by bank loan. My interview for 'Willesee at Seven' completed (I appealed for beds and an air-conditioner for Anthony) I prepared to sleep on cushions on the floor. No night light was set up, but candles instead. June, bless her, had not missed a thing off my list. I lit a candle and approached Anthony, standing forlornly by the electric fire. I had tried to explain we were going back to Australia, travelling in an aeroplane, to prepare him for so dramatic a change, but even after such a journey he expected his bedroom in the cottage back again. He whispered, 'Challock Lees, Mummy, back again.' By now the lights of Gawler were visible through the window topped by a bright crescent moon and a cluster of blue-white stars. 'Canterbury,' said Anthony. 'No darling,' I replied.

'It is Gawler; remember Mummy said we were going in an aeroplane, back to Australia?'

'Beautiful moon,' he sighed.

'Yes, my lamb, and sunshine tomorrow.'

'Sunshine, tomorrow,' he repeated. The cot was high and unpadded. 'Come sleep, little fellow, and I'll sing to you,' I coaxed. This hospital cot was from Estcourt House, an annexe of the Adelaide Children's Hospital. It was similar to the one in Kent, except the legs were not sawn off and the bars much lower. The candlelight was familiar and I held his hand and stroked his head until I thought my little traveller asleep. I spaced out the settee cushions on the floor and flung a sheet and blanket over them. I had just settled my aching body on to the ridges when Anthony said, 'God Bless Mummy. Go, Mummy!' Used to having, and sleeping in, his own room, I was dismissed! In a daze, gathering my dishevelled cushions and linen, I retreated to the kitchenette to fall asleep with my head beneath the sink and my feet against the stove.

The next day, like a broken doll, I lay scattered on the kitchen floor. Disorientated, I gathered up my pieces to answer Anthony's call. The cockerel was strutting on the gate outside the kitchen window, blasting its cock-a-doodle-do's to Daisy the cow, mooing in company; the ducks were quacking and the dogs were barking at the ducks and Anthony was yelling. Such a cacophony of sound, I thought I was dreaming. But staring at the sink, and down at the floor and the dead mosquitos I had kaputed in the night, I realised where I was.

June and Tony were leaving for work, and Mandy for school at seven. Our day had begun. It was warm and sunny and Anthony explored the fly wired porch and I lifted him up to see the strutting white cockerel, with his red magnificent head and his white entourage, picking and pecking their way up the yard. That afternoon, I managed to coax Anthony out into the sunshine to see the aviary of budgerigars. June, mother and Tony had checked the lawn as thoroughly as possible for painful three-cornered jacks, as I knew Anthony would still be bare-footed. He appeared quite happy, laughed at the rainbow of birds, raced around the lawn and even stripped off to run in and out of the spray from the sprinkler.

Our joy was short-lived. The bush flies, black obscenities, homed in to settle on the blood-scratched eczema. It was intolerable for him. They adhered and would not waft off. We had to return inside. I had problems during the day feeding Anthony as I just couldn't manage to crisp his toast the way he usually ate it. It was Vienna bread and I was not aware, at this stage, that Anthony was allergic to milk. He refused the toast.

That evening I prepared to bath him in the unit. The rest of the family were in the main part of the house. We were alone and we felt alone. Even though it was quite warm Anthony wanted the glow of the electric fire. I could hear the television and the movement through the walls, but Anthony and I were at the window, gazing at the deep purple sky and the myriads of stars crowning the glow of night lit, distant Gawler and, in between, the black ghostly silhouette of the gum trees and the slow-moving shadows of sheep. His allergy and the heat had dried Anthony's skin to lizard texture. With much coaxing I bathed him and coated him with a medicated form of petroleum jelly. It was difficult to hold him and I couldn't subject him to clothes.

Fatigue defeated him late into the evening and I placed him, tiny, naked and bald, into the rectangle of bars. 'Back again, Mummy, back to Challock Lees,' he cried. I lit a candle, placing it in a safe spot and kissed my son. The rising hysteria quelled as he lay staring at the swaying, soothing flame and fell asleep. I settled on the kitchen floor and stared out at the bright moon and stars, fascinated by their clarity.

It was so rare in Kent to see such a cloudless sky, such a view of distant worlds. And what of our world, I wondered? How would the Appeal fare in my absence? Would my supporters forget me? What is left for my little son? It was all happening, as I predicted. He had reached the end of his road. Tonight I could see again the haunted, yet strangely wild look of defeat in his eyes, as if he yearned for life yet cursed its cruelty; welcomed death yet spurned it. I wanted so much for my son and I always seemed to fail him.

The days ticked by. The sun tried to blaze through a dust storm but was dulled copper as the red-brown dust rose to obscure the skies. Hot and dry, I felt the world was on fire. I closed up the unit and played records to Anthony and felt as I had on that night of the storm in Challock ... wild, fearless, challenging. If this red glow was the end of the world, again I was ready; we were ready, my son and I.

Then the blood poured and Anthony bled everywhere, in competition with the world outside. He painted the unit red. My attempts to stop the flow were futile. For hours he bled and we revolved in a sea of red, a dance of suffering. Then it ceased, and exhausted, he lay snuffling on the bed. I placed my head in the nest of his chest and stomach and whispered, 'I love you, little man.' What had I done? My guilt was now overpowering. Would it have been better to have left him in Kent? Curled together, we fell asleep.

* * *

Two weeks passed and we had not left the unit. We were now in a new prison but, at least, mother was free. She happily gardened by day and joined the family at night.

That second Sunday a car screeched to a halt in a trail of dust. It was Anthony's father. Ted hadn't seen his son for over one and a half years. They did not know each other. Ted, however much he tried to conceal it, was horrified and Anthony was now indifferent. He had waited too long for his Daddy to return.

Anthony curled up on my bed. I played taped stories to him from the South Australian Education Department, who were wonderful in their approaches to help Anthony. I played 'The Woo Wind,' 'Snip, Snip and Snap,' 'The Old Kettle', and he lay and listened to the stores from a world of which he had not been allowed to be a part.

Anthony stopped eating completely and, after three weeks, wizened, worn, bleeding, his ribcage sticking out like leaf fronds, sore-eyed, he curled in his cot and refused to come out. When I tried to lift him, he whimpered as if my fingertips were barbs. I sat on the floor by his cot, sang quietly to him and held his delicate, lovely hand and realised the end had come. I didn't even know where we were. I was a stranger to this area. I felt as lost as my son and I bowed my head to my knees in submission.

Three days passed and Anthony stayed in his cot, refusing to drink or eat. I had already written to Anthony's neurosurgeon, who had saved his life almost six years previously. In desperation I phoned the Adelaide Children's Hospital and spoke with a doctor in the Department of Child and Family Psychiatry. He said he would come out to the farm the next day.

Anthony, as I predicted, had lost the will to live and, in all honesty, so had I. Did he reflect me or I him? Anthony was admitted to Estcourt House, by the sea, and he had a large playroom and a large bedroom. Five more days passed. Anthony still did not eat. I asked how long he could last and was told a week at the most. My sister-in-law, June, contacted Ted and he came to see Anthony, and after that visit came as often as he could. I was visited that day by two church ministers. One I did not know but the other I knew well … Tim, a former teaching colleague.

In my room we prayed together for Anthony and Tim said, 'Shirley, last night I had a vision of Anthony. His hair will regrow. I saw him quite clearly. He will not die here.' In my room in the now empty, original Estcourt House, a magnificent old stone doctor's residence bequeathed to the Children's Hospital, I stared at the beautiful domed, carved ceiling and screamed, 'No, Lord, no, not now!' I paced the majestic rooms, unafraid of the dark, the winding staircase leading high into the long-deserted servants' quarters.

Pacing like a ghost those lofty halls, I spoke aloud to myself, alone, struggling with self and my will for my son to live.

At dawn I went down to the ward with a new determination. As I nursed Anthony on my lap the morning sun threw light directly on to his pitiful bald head. I saw a halo, a down of fine gold hair. When I turned him out of the light it was not visible, so fine was the growth.

Anthony's hair was regrowing just as Tim had said. I talked to him, then sang to him. I don't remember the exact words; it is not important. Only the tone was important ... resolute, willing him to live. Whether Anthony sensed our fight was on again, whether the dedication of two special nurses worked, or the earnest prayers of Kathy and her group, and mother, I don't know.

But next morning, Anthony took a little food for the first time in over three weeks – with two days to live. I thanked God. We had caught the last embers of his life. That same morning Kathy came, bringing gifts of fruit and flowers. Barely able to see, she somehow finds her way around Australia helping others. I said, 'Kathy, he's had some food this morning.'

'Oh, I know,' she replied. 'Our prayer group gathered for a night vigil for him.' Kathy and those unknown friends prayed all through the night for Anthony and, from their prayers, unwearied, she came to be with us. I felt humbled. How could I have thought of giving in when strangers could join our struggle, body and soul? Mother arrived shortly afterwards, strangely elated. She was not unduly surprised by the good news, either. Staying with a friend in North Adelaide, she had awoken early, roused Doreen and said she would like to go to morning Mass. Doreen is a Catholic. The last time mother was in church, with feeling, was to christen my brother Tony twenty-six years before. At seven a.m. they went to Mass in a little church in Stanley Street and mother prayed as she had never prayed before.

On December 2, Anthony's sixth birthday, weighing less than 10 kilos, he had a party for the first time with other children. His

Daddy came and brought him a lovely fire engine for his birthday. Anthony was too ill to appreciate it, but I was warmed by the gesture. Hundreds of cards and telegrams flooded in from all over Australia. Toys and beautiful baskets of fresh fruit were sent and calls came in even from across the world to ask about Anthony and wish him joy on his birthday.

An Adelaide lady sent him a lovely ice-cream cake. He would not eat it but it made a splendid cake to share with the other patients. Anthony was so tiny he was lost in a baby's highchair, which was padded to support him. The kitchen staff had prepared lovely party foods but Anthony glanced, disinterested, at the feast, at the balloons and party hats and at the toot of party blowers. There was a reaction only when his birthday candles were lit. As he stared, and I stared at their reflection in his eyes, his gaze moved slowly about the room as the little ones and staff sang 'Happy Birthday to You, Happy Birthday dear Anthony' ... He was too weak to blow out the candles. It was done for him and everyone cheered. Bless the staff, they worked so hard to make it a happy birthday.

Now the tide was on the turn. It was my desire to stay with Anthony every moment but, again, it was felt that I was too strong an influence on him, that perhaps he would take other foods and respond more if I was absent. I was allowed only one hour visiting a day. I had to comply with the experiment as I had in the London hospital.

I was lost without my son. I conducted interviews or sat on the beach, and for the first time in my life, burnt to a blister as I sank deep in recriminations and forgot the unremitting sun. I swam for the first time in years. I had always been a beach and sun girl in the Mediterranean. Now, feeling old and tired, I was still able to sigh at the pleasure of the cool blue sea and the warm white sand.

When visiting, I brought what was left of my son down to the beach to the sea and waded with him, thigh deep, in the gentle waves but he hid his face from the sun in the nest of my shoulder and refused to look at the sea. Through my sadness I remembered back to those days in England when he would eagerly race to meet the waves in his gumboots and fisherman pants. Where was that lost child now? Even the spirit of the sea could not generate reaction.

The experiment was a failure. Without me, Anthony deteriorated again and developed pneumonia. Now I firmly refused to leave him and he was transferred to the Adelaide Children's Hospital. The wheel had truly come full circle. The same paediatrician who, at the foot of my bed, told me of Anthony's brain haemorrhage, the same ward, Princess, even some of the same kind sisters and nurses.

Anthony was put into Reece's room. Reece had shared the room with Anthony in the early days. He was a beautiful boy of 10, who just appeared to be permanently, peacefully, sleeping. His condition was a rare and ghastly side effect of measles. He was tube-fed through the nose, turned and washed and massaged and never once did I see him open his eyes. I was moved to think of the story of Sleeping Beauty in reverse ... that a princess's kiss might one day awaken him. His parents would come and sit by him, stroking his hair and holding his limp hand, but he was apparently unaware they were there. I could still see him as he was then, a beautiful sleeping statue.

This was where it had all begun six years ago. Anthony had returned. His lungs had to be gently pounded free of congestion and his painful cough eased.

Christmas, 1977, saw Anthony's hospital stocking at the foot of his bed. I had my room in the mothers' unit and spent Christmas Eve with Anthony and re-joined him early on Christmas morning. Ted came and blew balloons for Anthony and we were a family again for a little while sharing our only Christmas Day together since Anthony's first birthday. And Anthony was happy.

Now he improved. Mother and I were with him most of the day. I stayed until I tucked him into his cot and kissed him goodnight, heard his calm and secure, 'God Bless, Mummy, see you in the morning, when the sunshine comes.' The adjacent cubicle, the one in which Anthony had spent the first six months of his life, was empty. I was pleased that we were not in that end cubicle. As Anthony had a window he could see the babies through the glass.

A young boy in his mid-teens was admitted with advanced leukaemia. His name was Andrew. His mother and father were with him constantly. He was a very fortunate boy to have such wonderful parents. His father, a schoolteacher, humbled me by his example. Always bright, always a cheery smile, a wave and time to spare for Anthony. Our two families became very close. Anthony called him Rip; his name was Rick. The parents had known for three years that one day it would come to this and, in their love and courage, had kept it from their son. They had planned to return to England so that Andrew could see his grandparents and other members of the family for the first time, but the unpredictable disease rampaged and the grandparents came to their grandson.

One favourite song of Anthony's is 'The Londonderry Air' and mother told me that while she sang 'Oh, Danny Boy' "to Anthony the old couple joined in, stroking Andrew's head as he was slipping away. Those wonderful grandparents, singing to their dying grandchildren. They shared their vigils, sitting together as the two cubicles became one. They crooned all the old songs that old as I am, I am too young to remember. I only learned of it afterwards, when Anthony survived and left hospital, and mother told me the full story.

One day I arrived after Anthony's nap for my half of the day to find him still asleep and Andrew's room empty. I had said goodnight to him at 9.30 the previous evening, leaving him sitting holding his father's hand as they watched television.

'You'll soon be going home.' I said. 'You look so well.' 'Yes,' he said, 'goodnight, I'll see you tomorrow.' Now it was tomorrow.

'Where's Andrew?' I asked.

'He's gone,' said the nurse. I thought he'd gone home, in a brief moment of optimism, but he had died at eleven o'clock that morning, speedily.

Anthony knew ... I'm sure he knew. The kind nurse had tried to coax Anthony out of Andrew's room, but he stayed until the door was closed on him and five minutes later Andrew died.

At the end of the ward were the two cubicles I knew so well. I placed a chair opposite the two doors and stared first at Anthony, asleep, and *CLICK* ... six years into the past I saw Reece, now dead, then stared into the empty cubicle which had been Andrew's last home. I could see him laughing, hand-linked with his father, alive, but now where was he? My head sank to my knees. Silently, the chirpy young physiotherapist coughed and made me raise my head. She had come to massage Anthony's lungs but he was still asleep: Why, I sighed? After all these years I still could not accept or understand. What a lovely family they were; his brave mother and loving grandparents and his father, who bathed him, fed him and, until his last second on earth, loved and supported him. If only every child could die with such love.

One day a few weeks later we all met again in Tea-Tree Plaza. Anthony wanted to jump on the escalator as we greeted each other like family. The old couple were returning to England, and Rick was taking leave and he and his wife were going with them. They still had a smile, words of encouragement and a kiss for Anthony. They were such truly remarkable parents. I shall never forget them.

Chapter 19

Between Christmas and New Year my former next-door neighbour, Erica, came to visit with news that our old house was empty. She'd seen the owners and it was to let. She asked if I was interested. As Anthony had been growing stronger I knew I had to plan our future. We could not return to the farm; it was too isolated and dusty following the winter's drought. After all the effort, love and care of my family to try to make a home for us, how could I tell them we would not be returning? I definitely wanted to rent our old home.

Erica arranged a meeting and I entered the empty house, paid a month's rent in advance, received the keys and the owners left. I walked the empty rooms, so familiar, the same carpets, the same curtains, the same wallpaper; only the furniture was missing, gone with the past five years of our lives. I opened the pantry door and still clearly visible were the first months of Anthony's life I had marked off, awaiting his death, before the news of the first transplant and the long years past in England. I now had my home back, even if it was not, literally, mine. I had wonderful neighbours and there were lots of children for Anthony to play with.

Having seen Rick make his dying son happy I vowed Anthony would be happy for as long as God allowed. I would isolate him no longer.

The carpets were steam-cleaned to kill germs and repainted the interior of the house. I hosed the exterior and disinfected under sills and steps for redback, poisonous spiders. By the New Year all was ready. My tenancy officially began on New Year's Day. June gave me her old lounge suite. We had been given beds and wardrobes; we had all we needed. Everyone was so kind. On New Year's Eve I left the hospital at ten p.m. 'God Bless, Anthony, I'll see you next year and whatever 1978 holds for you,' I said, 'may it be happiness.'

Erica and Paul next door had planned a New Year's Eve party and I arrived to the hearty greeting of old friends, good food, wine, music and laughter. The sounds over the fence of the splash of neighbours into their pools highlighted the life of it all. I tipped back a glass of cool white wine, my face raised to the stars, and breathed the warmth of human contact. I was home at last.

* * *

That first day-night of 1978, after the party, I had but a few steps to go to my bedroom. I flicked on the light switch and looked at what had been mine and Ted's bedroom. My single bed made the room appear even larger.

In the darkness, propped high on my pillows, I could see the swaying shapes of the trees we had planted together with such love, planning a future. Would it have been a different ending if I hadn't taken Anthony to London? As a welcome cool draught filtered through the fly screens I sighed in unison. Who knows? I did what had to be done and I had no regrets.

This was my first night in a bed of my own for weeks. I had slept in hard hospital beds and now I rolled in the luxury of its softness and reflected on events since our return to Australia. It had nearly proved a disastrous move. I had almost lost Anthony. At our lowest ebb, when again I desperately called for help, it had not been in vain.

Due to an odd mixture of caring by medical staff, prayer groups, family, friends and strangers, another strained circle had been full drawn. I was back in the room where I had prayed so earnestly that Good Friday, 1973, for life for Anthony. And he was still alive this new day of 1978. I was planning a new life for him and soon he would be well enough to join me and return to his own room. It was exactly as he had left it, only newly painted, the same patterned curtains, a little faded now, and his metal cot instead of his beautiful carved wooden one.

It was mid-January when, released from hospital, looking like a little convict with his stubble of new hair, he sat on his Nanna's lap and stared at the house as I turned into the drive and stopped the car in the shade of the carport. Would he recognise his home? Would another change trigger those horrifying battering sessions? Would he shut himself away again as he had at the farm? All these questions and more flashed through my mind as I walked round the car to lift him out. He hadn't been upset when the car stopped, he didn't resist when I lifted him out and into the house and he smiled as he looked about him. He struggled, signalling his desire to be put down, and began exploring the rooms. He sensed it was his sole domain and he had his Nanna and Mummy back again.

It was accepted and that evening he positioned himself without fuss at the end of the hallway to run down to his room. 'On my mark, ready, set, go,' he said and my frail little Anthony tottered down to his room and I caught him and swung him into his cot. There was no padding. I'd decided this had to be. It was not needed. Anthony's new lifestyle had begun. No more isolations. Neighbours and their children were free and welcome to walk in and out. The lounge looked like a play school with toys and children everywhere. Anthony would tolerate them for a little while and then the noise and excitement became too much. It was a gradual process, this acceptance of bouncing, normal children. They expected him to respond and accept their invitations to play and he couldn't. He didn't know how.

He had never played with children before, but little Natalie came to his aid. Erica's pretty three-year-old from next door, like a mother hen, took Anthony under her wing and spoke quietly and gently to him. She brought all her favourite toys to show him – her doll Jill-Pill, her pram, her carry-basket and musical TV set and, never having parted with any before, allowed Anthony to 'borrow' them.

This was the start of their friendship. She was Anthony's first friend. He called her Natnat. She came in the morning, sometimes still in her pyjamas and slippers, and shared his toast and 'gob'. It took me quite a while to work out Natalie's 'gob'; it was Bovril. It was astounding, the understanding of a three-year-old like Natalie of Anthony's needs. At first she allowed him to take everything he wanted. It was a great sacrifice to lose her rows of beautiful, coloured beads and her high-heeled slippers.

I was pleased when their relationship reached a stage where Anthony understood sharing for the first time. I blew bubbles for them. They each had a wand and, in turn, caught a bubble and burst it. Anthony wanted all the bubbles. Hadn't they always been all his bubbles? 'These are for Natalie and these are for Anthony,' I repeated again and again. He learned. If Natalie had a toy he, at first, took it. No one had ever questioned this taking in his adult world. They had never wanted his toys. Now began the teaching of being a part of a world. He had to learn that he should share his toys, and he did.

I went to our local primary school and saw the headmistress – a vibrant, kind, understanding woman – and arranged to take Anthony to school each day as an experiment. It was planned he should join one class to try to identify with a specific teacher and classmates. Those first few days of Anthony's freedom still found me instinctively looking and listening for coughs and colds and wondering if any of the children were sickening for mumps or measles.

'You have to stop this, Shirley ... You have made a decision and there are no half measures. Take each day as it comes and make it as normal and happy as possible for Anthony,' I spoke again to my inward self.

The first day of school we arrived late. Anthony's morning routine was still very slow, being so used to endless days and endless time. He joined his class and teacher, looked fearlessly around, then left the unit and set out to explore the rest of the school. I had noted again the mixed reactions of the children. Like the adults on the plane there was fear, revulsion, interest and compassion. Dragging me along, Anthony discovered the play school. This was to be his favourite room for the first weeks of term. He called it the 'Hey-diddle-diddle' room because from the ceiling were suspended life-sized coloured shapes relating to the nursery rhyme. Each time we entered the room he recited that nursery rhyme. He carefully avoided the toddlers pounding their play dough, using their creative talents in paste-paint, laughing or crying, intent on their various pursuits. He barely glanced as he meandered among them and they backed away, staring at the strange little figure, still patchy bald, thin, pale and marked with eczema. He found his way out into the wide outdoor play area. He simply liked to stand there alone and listen to the hubbub inside as if he wanted to get used to it. He didn't wish to join them and did not respond to the approach of the inevitable demonstrative or friendly toddler who came to make friends. He would occasionally spare a word, shyly, for Miss Sandy or Miss Williams.

He explored the main primary school building, an Aladdin's Cave, blue-carpeted, open-plan designed. Areas were sectioned off by the children's own work. Things like an Indian Reserve, a flower display, an animal, fish, bird or car collection. There were play areas, work areas, a music room, art-work sections and letters, numbers and colours creating a fascinating children's world. Anthony wandered round observing but not communicating. Most of the children knew who he was and had some idea that he had been very, very ill, but children can be so honest.

'Yuk,' said one little boy as we passed. I found the same mixed response as I took Anthony to St Agnes shopping centre. Those who recognised us eagerly, or shyly, came and greeted us, to wish us well. It was very difficult for Anthony, unused as he was to the world, to have these kind, but huge, strange, smiling faces thrust at him saying, 'Hello, Anthony, how are you?' He didn't reply but tugged at my hand to explore further. The music and the bright lights of the complex fascinated him. I let him wander about at will, then decided to try an experiment. I was going to take Anthony shopping for the first time. I pushed through the turnstyle and coaxed Anthony to follow. He tugged, instead of pushed, and confused, shook it. Angry, he solved his problem by crawling underneath. We wandered up and down as I pointed out things he knew, like fruit and vegetables, bread, packets of cereal, aisle by aisle until we reached the toy section at the end. I carried just a loaf of bread so that I could handle Anthony. He examined everything until he came to a container of multi-coloured beachballs. He wrestled and tugged until he grasped a huge ball, barely managing to hold it in the circle of his arm. 'But you have one at home,' I said, then stopped my argument in midstream. This was Anthony's first shopping expedition. He had chosen his purchase. 'Come on little fellow, let's pay the lady,' I said. I turned away and walked to the end of the aisle, assuming Anthony was following; but he had retraced his steps to the bin of balls. He was struggling with another.

'I want two,' he said. At $1.58 each, I thought, Anthony didn't understand about money.

'If you can carry two you can take two,' I said. 'Mummy has to carry the bread.' He struggled fruitlessly to hold the second one. The two balls bounced down the aisle. He tried again and again but could only manage one. I placed the other back in the bin and, quite happily, two hands now rimming the one bright ball, he said, 'Pay the lady, Mummy.'

I didn't bargain for the attraction of the revolving counter when I placed the loaf on it and it moved. 'Oh again, Mummy, again,' he said. So I placed the loaf at the end and the co-operative and amused check-girl made it move once again. I showed Anthony the dollars and cents. I paid the lady at Anthony's request and spent quite a while coaxing him away from the check-out by the promise of a game with his new ball.

The next day at the school and the 'Hey-diddle-diddle' room there was the same behaviour till, turning to leave, Anthony said, 'Let's go to pay the lady.' At the supermarket again he battled the turn-style and, in defeat, crawled underneath. He tugged me up and down the aisles looking earnestly to right and left. At first I thought he was just curious, but he showed his determination to continue parading up and down even after I'd picked up the bread and showed it to him and said, 'I'll pay the lady now.' 'No, Mummy,' he said, and tugged away. We went on again. Then I realised he was looking for the toy section so I guided him there. Releasing my hand he made it directly to the bin of beach balls, scooped one out, identical to yesterday's, propped it under his arm and marched back to me, a look of satisfaction on his face. 'Pay the lady, Mummy,' he said. He looked so happy that I swallowed my reasoning and realised I had a lot of teaching to do before tomorrow's 'pay the lady' day. That evening we played with the identical beach balls in the lounge. The next morning I took them in the car with us.

Before we went shopping I pointed to the balls on the back seat. 'You have two,' I said. 'No more today, Anthony.' He understood and instead headed for the lolly aisle and picked a packet of brightly coloured liquorice allsorts. He doesn't eat them but he likes to use them as mini-building blocks.

Within a month Anthony had a new vocabulary and new confidence. I could take him alone in the car. He says, 'Start the engine, Mummy,' and, as it is an atrocious starter, he yells, 'Fingers crossed, Mummy,' jumping up and down in his seat till the engine roars to life.

Off we would drive to school, to Miss Meredith's class, on to the supermarkets, the bank, the delicatessens, until, slowly, a bright new world was opening before him. Each morning he eagerly asked to go to school. He visited his own class and laughed, enjoyed the children singing and playing number games, wandered to the play school, then into the blue room, as Anthony named the main school. He discovered a number wheel and a large teaching clock and I taught him to recognise the symbols for the numbers he could already count. He also quickly learned one to 12 o'clock.

I was delighted; he learned so rapidly. But he would not join the other children and, usually, rejected any approaches by teachers. We stayed as long as Anthony wanted and I allowed him to explore at will. He had a lot to make up.

Chapter 20

The routine strengthened Anthony; his days are now full and exciting, not monotonous and empty. He's mastered the turnstyle at the supermarket, helps push my trolley, has learned to queue at the check-out, carries my shopping, wanders in and out of other shops and even tells the lady in the chemist that her light has broken.

He has become quite a familiar little figure, especially in the post office. I tried a new experiment by allowing him to post my letters. I lifted him up to the post box but he wanted to keep the letters. I stood on one side, holding him at the height of the slit, as others posted their mail. I told him that we had to put the letters in the box for the postman to fill his bag to put them through letterboxes. The postman in Challock Lees had been a close friend and Anthony understood about letters coming through the door and plopping on the mat. He posted the letters. The next day it was successful, but the third day I had problems – no letters! Anthony stood crying by the post box, real tears. I was astounded. Anthony often yelled and screamed but so rarely cried. I dashed into the post office and collected some leaflets. Our little drama had been witnessed by my friends behind the counter. I lifted Anthony up to post the letters and, inside, the chap put his hand into the post box so that when Anthony posted a letter a hand took it. He was entranced. It gave me quite a start at first. When he tried to post his last leaflet the hand pushed it back again. Anthony was chuckling with glee, trying to push the leaflet past the active fingers. I think I gave in first and lowered Anthony to the pavement. 'More tomorrow,' I said, and turned crimson at the amused crowd of spectators waiting to post their mail.

Our regular visits to the post office at St Agnes set a pattern until Anthony had to enter the shopping complex via the post office whether I needed stamps or not.

The next step was to try Anthony at the larger shopping complex in the area, Tea-Tree Plaza. I parked in the large arrowed parking lanes, lifted Anthony out and steered him to the entrance. At St Agnes he had been fascinated by the parking arrows on the bitumen. Dodging cars, we explored the parking lines and arrows. 'They're cracked and faded,' said Anthony in disgust. 'Well, I have a surprise for you,' I replied. The large brown brick complex looked uninteresting. 'This building,' I said, 'has magic doors; we say, "open sesame" and they open by themselves. We don't even have to push them.' We approached the entrance and within a few yards of the automatic doors they glided open. Anthony looked at my hands then looked at his, quite puzzled. We walked into the first arcade and, swoosh, the door closed behind us. As Anthony turned to look and examine this phenomenon the doors opened and we were again outside. 'Open sesame,' said Anthony. In and out, out and in, the sideways glares of shoppers displaying suppressed amusement. Tiring of the game, or satiated by the experience, we continued into the complex. We examined each shop until we reached the centre area where the kiddi-cars are placed. Ladybird, the roundabout, bucking-horses, bumping cars, coaches, fire engines, swaying rockets and motor-trucks. Anthony stood watching the speeding, squealing, happy children then continued his mission of exploration.

He rapidly discovered the escalator. All or nothing, I thought. 'Up the hill, Anthony, ready, steady, go,' I said. He mastered it immediately and laughed with abandoned happiness as we glided upwards and turned his head this way and that, drinking in the wine of lights, movement and people, Ladybirds spinning below and the escalator gliding down opposite. 'Ready to jump, Anthony,' I said, and swirled him off to explore the top shopping area. He headed for the spotlights of the display area, examined them thoroughly then discovered the TV rental shop. 'Twenty together,' he said. I'd only taught him to count to 20 and he encompassed the silent, coloured, animated TV sets in his outstretched arms.

Going down the escalator was more of a problem. Anthony wanted the run of the hill to himself. I had to stall him until it was clear.

This is how our days revolved until I had allowed him to explore all of his environment, within reason and safety, and Anthony had proved more than equal to the challenge. We had our problems at weekends. On the first Saturday, Anthony wanted to go to school. Each day had been the same for Anthony for six years; how could he comprehend Saturday? I drove him to school and we wandered around the deserted buildings, Anthony peering in this window and that. 'Nobody's there, darling,' I said. 'Nobody here,' he echoed, and Sunday was the same. This continued until the headmistress heard and gave me a key to Anthony's classroom. So now he goes to school seven days a week.

The next experiment was to take mother to my brother's farm. She spent each weekend with them, sharing her time between our two families. Usually she travelled up by bus or train. As we turned off on to the dirt road to the farm Anthony looked about him. I stopped at the farm gate, closed because Whisky the horse was loose grazing, climbed out, opened the gate, drove through a few yards, climbed out and closed it. Anthony said not a word; he was quietly observing all. I was apprehensive that he may think he was being brought back here to stay. Lady, the Doberman, came snapping round the car and Kovash, the old basset hound, hollowly coughed. June came out and locked the dogs in the yard. Without hesitation, Anthony clambered out and looked about him.

He wouldn't go into the house but he did walk the half kilometre down the drive to inspect the gate. Back in the car he said, 'Fetch Nanny now.'

'No, she's staying with Auntie June and will come back again tomorrow,' I explained. I waved goodbye and drove off. Now, each Saturday, Anthony says, 'Go to see Lady and open the gate.'

Preparations were underway at school, although Anthony took no part, in the making of Easter bunnies, painting eggs or learning songs for parents' night. Anthony decided he wanted to go into the blue school. All the children were assembled, seated on the carpeted activity area. The piano burst forth with 'Easter Bunny' and then 'In Your Easter Bonnet', to the accompaniment of a hundred or so enchanting voices, in key and out, backed by their various expressions of joy, concentration and mischief. It was eyes left as we approached and the voices faltered for an instant. I sat on the carpet beside the children with Anthony on my lap. The headmistress rallied the rehearsal with force over the intercom. Staff, children and I sang with gusto. I have never seen Anthony look happier. 'I want it again,' he called. With abandon the children laughed but the piano beat out 'In Your Easter Bonnet', and Anthony clapped in unison. The rehearsal over, the children filed out to morning break but Anthony remained 'Seated on my knee. 'Want "In Your Easter Bonnet" again, Mummy,' he said. In the car, in the supermarket and at home I sang the song over and over again as Anthony clapped, listened and then joined in.

Miss Williams had informed me that at 9. 30 the next morning she would hold the final rehearsal for parents' evening. It was the earliest I ever managed to get Anthony to school. The whole primary school assembled and sang their songs, some dramatised, and I remembered my own days rehearsing my children for the Christmas pantomimes and Nativity plays, and with amazement I realised that we were experiencing a day I never thought would be possible – Anthony was sitting with his contemporaries at school and joining in the singing. I was bursting with joy.

The next day I ambled up the path to school. Anthony by-passed his unit, by-passed the 'Hey-diddle-diddle' room and made straight for the main school. To his disappointment the activity area was empty. The blue carpet stretched away, a flat, uninteresting ocean. The children were busy at their lessons. Undeterred, Anthony sat down and waited. 'In Your Easter Bonnet,' he said. 'It's finished,' I explained. 'It was for Easter and Easter's gone.' He didn't understand; he waited and waited until, with resignation, he left the building and trudged down the path to the car. He hasn't returned to the blue-carpeted room.

Anthony could now find his way about the school and he had ceased to be a curiosity. His hair had re-grown and his eczema was more controlled. He was now accepted. His classmates, lovely kids, greeted him each time he arrived and Anthony would tolerate, but not communicate with them. Gradually they stopped crowding him and the release of pressure enabled him to relax more.

I loved being with the children again and they called me Auntie Shirley. One little boy said, 'When Anthony first came I thought he was sort of yukky weird.'

'I don't blame you,' I said. 'He is a strange little fellow but he's had a tough time, you know.'

'Oh, I do know,' the lad replied. 'Now I know him, I think he's terrific.'

'Indeed he is,' I smiled.

Chapter 21

Anthony was still the size of a three-year-old and his six- or seven-year-old classmates were a little amazed when he counted, sang or recited for them, or joined their games on some of the rare occasions he stayed long enough to do more than be fascinated by the fans revolving to cool the air.

The school holidays loomed for two whole weeks and I was worried the break in our routine would disrupt Anthony; that he'd wonder about the empty school, thinking that all the children had deserted him, as adults always did. Each day of the two-week holiday I took Anthony to school. He accepted this and the Sunday before the new term I told him the girls and the boys would be back again the next day.

Now Anthony only went into his own unit. He had ceased to explore the rest of the school. Sometimes he stayed a few minutes only. Sometimes he would join in a song, paint a picture or play with a classmate, talk to Miss Jo, a new teacher, then abruptly close off and say, 'To the post office!'

After two terms we had taken but a tiny step into Anthony's new world but he was already reading his first words. Only six months out of isolation, he enjoyed visitors, children and adults. He knew the area in which we lived, the journeys south to the city and north to Gawler, and he had two special friends, Bugs Bunny and Natalie – one a toy and one real.

He began to talk to Bugs Bunny, his first break from reality, and to faithful, beautiful Natalie, who accompanied us, whenever possible, to school and to the farm. She washed Anthony's back in his bath, rubbed his wet hair, even helped to empty his potty and treat his eczema. 'Nurse Byrne' I have dubbed her, this compassionate three-year-old. She was allowed more privileges than I with my little son. She decided that she was going to marry him.

Each week Ted called to say 'hello' and have a game, or to take Anthony for a ride around the creek in his pushchair. One day, on our way to school, Anthony picked two flowers, yellow soursops bright as the winter sunshine. He handed them to two pretty girls in his class. They were delighted and so was I. That gesture of giving flowers, from one child to another, was Anthony's first real reaching out. He was now responding to their approaches, a big step for one little boy, new in a very large world.

The next day the blood flowed again for the first time in eight months, a stream he breathed and swallowed until he choked and coughed it out, a crimson impression of the past seven years.

I realised how little had changed, looking at the sore, white and bloodied face of my son and his little body heaving intermittently with the aftermath of sobs.

I wiped the blood from the floor. Pushing back my hair, I inadvertently wiped a red streak across my forehead – a mark of seven tragic years. I was back in the same house, having travelled the world, still drowning in the sea of my son's blood.

And I still would not accept that it had to be so.

* * *

In September 1978 I flew to London for a vision became reality – the official opening of the Anthony Nolan Laboratories. It was a wonderful day, meeting not only all my dear friends and allies from press, radio and TV, but also all the area organisers for the Appeal, a band of golden-hearted, hard-working, voluntary workers, without whose help our entire medical project would grind to a halt.

It was during this brief stay in London that Dr James outlined a programme of experiments being carried out by the transplant team. The idea was to manufacture a compatible donor for Anthony, from myself or Anthony's father, by a desensitising technique. No more was revealed at the time as the professors and doctors wished to conduct more tests. It did mean, however, that I carried within me a new glimmer of hope on my return to Australia and a directive to withdraw, once again, Anthony's supporting steroid drug.

Once the steroids had been withdrawn, the drug prednisolone drastically affected Anthony. His appetite waned and he lost weight rapidly. His eczema flared until his entire emaciated little body was raw, red and painful, with numerous infected sores. Antibiotics did not help at all.

I coaxed, even pleaded with him to eat, to no avail. I spent hours daily treating his skin with special baths and soothing ointments. His deterioration continued.

Valiant as ever, Anthony still asked to go to school, although we did little more than manage the walk up the path to his classroom, a brief 'hello' to the children, then back to the car. Now his favourite part of the day was a ride in the roundabout at Tea-Tree Plaza shopping precinct. He would grip the steering wheel tightly in this replica of a flying saucer, as it soared impressively high into the air, spiralling and hissing gaily.

Five minutes, ten minutes, sometimes as long as half an hour, he sat entranced, lost in his own little world – thinking who knows what? – as a kaleidoscope veered past him. We had to switch off the power to entice him out, and stiffly, clutching my hand, he hobbled back to the car.

'Tomorrow,' he sighed. 'More tomorrow.' For Anthony's seventh birthday I planned a party for all the 'Creek Kids'. There were balloons, party hats, ice-cream, cakes, presents and laughter. Anthony loved it, although he was too weak to join actively the crowd of bubbling, healthy kiddies. He was content to sit on my knee, unwrap his presents and light and blow out his birthday candles.

It was hard not to lose control and cry at the sight of my tiny seven-year-old with barely enough strength to extinguish the flames, as I realised that his life was now as tenuous as the light from those fragile candles.

Each morning Anthony's cot sheet, a witness to his night's suffering, was a collage of spattered blood and flecks of lacerated skin. His legs became painfully swollen and his feet so puffy that it was impossible even to put on loose sandals. He tried to walk, whimpering with pain; he wanted to go to his roundabout.

Pale and listless, he was always cold. Teeth chattering, he would ask to have the fire on. Incredibly, it was mid-summer and over 90° outside; yet Anthony would curl for warmth in my lap, on the floor in front of the fire or in the sunlight streaming through the French windows and fall asleep.

I looked at him and prayed, 'Dear Lord, if Anthony is meant to die, please let it be like this, peacefully at home.'

I had, of course, phoned London at intervals to report on Anthony's condition. This time when I dialled, I clutched the phone with trembling hands. I didn't know how far the professor had progressed with his experiments – we had planned not to return to London until spring to avoid influenza. With the withdrawal of steroids I had expected a deterioration in Anthony's condition, but not with such horrific swiftness. It was early in January 1979. Britain was suffering its worst winter for decades, but we could delay no longer or Anthony would be dead.

As I replaced the receiver, plans were set in train to return to London in a week's time. I then phoned Anthony's father, who came immediately to help plan the journey. He was full of enthusiasm and encouragement, yet I felt drained and dejected. I knew what lay ahead. I knew what had to be done. Hadn't we done it all before in 1973? But I was younger then, I mused, full of hope, and never in my wildest imaginings had I envisaged the turmoil and heartache of the ensuing six years.

I felt I couldn't go through it all again – the interminable flying hours, witnessing Anthony's pain and bewilderment, knowing the isolation and the complex tests to which he would be subjected.

Conflicting emotions surged one after another. Would I have carried on in 1973 if I had known the future? Wasn't I deluding myself that Anthony could even survive the gruelling journey, or that there was any guarantee that the tests would even work? Wouldn't it be kinder to readmit Anthony to the Adelaide Children's Hospital, sedate him, render him pain-free and let him die in peace? My God, hadn't he suffered enough?

The truth was that I didn't want to go through it all again. I felt utterly exhausted, physically and spiritually. I can't face it, I said to myself, I can't go on. And I knew mother felt the same. 'Dear God,' I cried out, 'dear God, give us strength.'

The next morning, at Anthony's call, I went to take him from his cot, but when I touched him he cried out in pain. He felt sticky. Apart from the blood, a thin yellowish fluid oozed from his skin, and with it an odour of rotting flesh. With disbelief, I stared at his scrotum, enlarged with fluid like a huge, finely veined pouch.

He couldn't straighten his limbs and I had to lift him, curled like a foetus. Gently I handed him to mother and called London. Mrs Marian Matthews, our Appeal secretary, was making the arrangements for our flight. I said that it was imperative we leave immediately. I sat anxiously by the phone until the early hours. With expertise and grim determination, Marian somehow organised everything. Her call confirmed our flight for the next day, and I rang to alert Ted, who was coming with us.

Departure time from Adelaide was 8 p.m. At 7 p.m. I still hadn't managed to dress Anthony. He cringed at the slightest touch. I had gently nursed him most of the day and had managed his bath. While he slept I flung a few essentials into my suitcase and filled Anthony's with his favourite toys. I despaired of even making the flight.

The suitcases were piled into the car of Jenny, my next-door neighbour; its engine ticked over, awaiting our departure. By now I was in my bedroom, sobbing. Erica, my other neighbour, came in and wept with me.

'I'll never manage it,' I said.

'Come on,' she said, 'you can do it. Just get our little man there.' Yes, I thought, I must. Somehow, in those final minutes, I dressed Anthony in a cotton shirt, loose pants and large socks. The car sped to the terminal, where we met Ted, and we boarded immediately, after a sad farewell to our neighbours and the 'Creek Kids', who had gathered in force.

I numbly registered Adelaide, Perth, Bombay, London – a thirty-hour journey during which I made a bed of my body for Anthony and kept as still as possible to save him pain. He never complained but clutched me grimly, lips taut. He asked me to sing to him, which I did continuously, one song after another, willing him to live.

The bump of wheels on tarmac – the icy blast of a -2° winter's dawn – the whirr and clank of the emergency air lift – a surge of Press and cameras – calls of good luck – the slam of ambulance doors – the familiar London buildings, blurred in the grey light, and the finality of walls around us in an isolation cubicle at Westminster Children's Hospital.

* * *

Anthony clung to me pathetically as gowned figures passed in and out. Little was done immediately; only the essential task of assessing expertly Anthony's present condition. Only when we were alone was I able to coax him out of his clothes, carefully easing off blood-soaked socks from his now massive, swollen legs, and finally his vest, yellow, soaked and skin-clotted.

I sang and soothed and gently bathed and creamed his skin until his pain eased a little. Mercifully, he slept, exhausted.

A consultation with the transplant professor and senior consultant paediatrician confirmed my fears: Anthony was oedematous, a condition caused by lack of protein, and in such an advanced state of deterioration that there was some doubt about whether he would now be able to absorb food at all. A feeding tube was inserted through his nose and into his stomach, down which a machine pumped dilute soya milk, a few millilitres an hour. Daily the amount and strength were increased. A week later Anthony's skin was dry, though still very sore. The odour had disappeared and the suppuration had ceased. His condition was further improved by transfusions of irradiated blood for his anaemia and platelets to prevent haemorrhaging. Special cream was applied to his head and body, and his arms and legs were plastered in thick coal-tar bandages.

Anthony's arms had to be fastened to splints and then to the cot bars. Although weak, he was angrily trying to wrench out the nasal-gastric tube. I had to reason with him daily that he could have his arms untied if he didn't touch his tube. Finally he agreed. Now he was furious at the restricting bandages. I was pleased. I could see a glint in his eye – his old fighting spirit was back again.

The tests to manufacture a donor now began. Blood was taken from Anthony, myself, Anthony's father and grandmother (my mother, wonderful as ever, also volunteered to be part of the experiment). In test tubes cells from each of us were mixed with Anthony's. As anticipated, Anthony's produced other cells to attack ours, and ours reacted in the same way. These cells were then carefully separated. Anthony's attacking cells were injected back into him and ours into us.

As these cells were produced outside our bodies, in test tubes, the theory was that our immunity systems would now treat them as alien cells, attack them and negate them. Thus, we would be 'switched off' and no attacking cells would remain.

We knew we were guinea pigs. The professor had carefully explained that there could be side effects and that he would only attempt these experiments on close relatives who were willing volunteers. We had no hesitation. The injections were given in each arm and each buttock – four in all. Then, a week later, another four. They were painful, like bee stings, and I cringed at the thought of Anthony's reaction to the same course of injections.

After blood tests, mother and Anthony's father still retained all their attacking cells, yet Anthony had 'switched off' to all three of us. He could now accept a bone marrow transplant from one of us. The only one left in the running was me.

After the first four injections I had 'switched off' enough attacking cells to be Anthony's donor. Tragically, after the second four injections (which, it is now realised, I did not need) my attacking cells reactivated and increased. In my case, another four injections were given in the hope that my cell count would drop again, but it rose even higher. We had failed.

The professor was as disappointed as we were. The chances looked so good. The reason he had pressed on was because of Anthony's critical condition. Our haste to help him lost me as his donor. I couldn't feel bitterness – only resignation. Where did we go from here? No donor, no transplant. I must confess that at the time it was only small consolation to have the professor's words ringing in my ears: 'We have, however, learnt a great deal more from these experiments and are now trying to help children from other families.'

The next proposed treatment was to infuse Anthony with some of his father's white cells. If this worked, it could give Anthony sufficient immunity to cope with day-to-day living for as long as four years. We would be buying time until the laboratories found the perfect donor.

On Monday, March 19th, over two months since our arrival, the infusion was ready and was dripped intravenously into Anthony's arm. It was an extremely difficult process, as his veins are worn or collapsed. The needle and splint caused him grave discomfort in the early stages, and towards evening his hand began to swell. The cells had gone into his tissue; the vein was blocked. The needle was re-sited, but the infusion tissued again and again, until Anthony was hysterical with pain. Ted was a great help that long evening, sitting with Anthony and helping Sister. We wanted to stay with him until the vital infusion was complete.

I sat in Sister's office, the room next to Anthony's, unable to alleviate his suffering but just wanting to be near him. If I had been in the room, he would have wanted to be in my lap instead of lying flat and keeping his arm straight and still.

The white cell infusion left his hand and arm hideously swollen and covered with white blisters as if he had been burnt.

My God, I thought, how much more does this little one have to take?

How could he possibly understand why we allowed so many strangers to hurt him? Blood tests, transfusions, complex dental surgery, splints, bandaged limbs, injections, tubes into his stomach and examination after examination, all by green-gowned and masked figures. All kind – but how intense his confusion, horror and sadness in his interminable isolation.

A few days later Ted left and returned to Adelaide. He believed the white cell infusion would work and we would be following shortly.

With disbelief I listened to the professor's report that it had not worked. There was no improvement at all in Anthony's immunity.

The final attempt to help Anthony was by the use of a drug called thymosin. It involved a daily injection for a week, then twice a week for at least six weeks, before any results would show. The drug was known to have helped 60 per cent of Wiskott-Aldrich Syndrome patients, from reports from America, both improving immunity and controlling the ghastly eczema.

Now we had to wait. Initially Anthony had adapted well to isolation and had several favourites amongst the nurses. He could instantly recognise them by their voice or eyes. But as the months passed, I could see again a haunted look in his eyes. He talked frequently of home, Natalie, his little girlfriend from next door, his roundabout, the shops, and often said: 'I'm going to school tomorrow.' It was impossible to explain just why he had to be locked away in a tiny room.

I began to worry about the side effects of his long isolation. I know how destructive it had been in the past, and I eagerly awaited the results of the thymosin treatment to see if it was possible to plan going home.

Our life in the hospital and mothers' unit again deeply affected mother and me. It is impossible to live in such close proximity with other mothers and not become personally involved. At times we were profoundly depressed when Anthony failed to respond to treatment, then a familiar face appeared from down the years and a warm reunion followed: Brenda with Tracey, now a bonny six-year-old in callipers; Jean and her son Francis, now eleven – both children victims of spina bifida. The same brave mums returning time and again, coping with one crisis after another.

There were also happy times, like when Richard Sharp, cured of leukaemia by a bone marrow transplant, was able to go home; when Caron, critically ill and haemorrhaging with leukaemia, finally went into remission and could also go home. Her name was added to the list on our laboratory wall of patients urgently needing a bone marrow donor.

Then followed the heartache of days like Easter Sunday.

I met Ann Storey when in London to open the Anthony Nolan Laboratories. Leanne, her pretty, bright-eyed baby girl, was kicking happily in her sterile plastic bubble. Her transplant was progressing well. Ann was still resident in the hospital when we returned in January and Leanne was able to play happily in her baby-walker up and down the ward.

Her first birthday was a great celebration, as they would soon be going home. Leanne then developed diarrhoea and began to vomit and lose weight rapidly. Ann came sobbing to our room with the news that Leanne was to be returned to her sterile bubble for a booster transplant. Her donor, Mrs Angela Harffy, was recalled.

The major problem was that apart from her immune deficiency, Leanne was born with a congenital heart defect. Ann became distraught as Leanne battled but became weaker and weaker. The strain on her heart was proving too much. Ann's mother arrived and my mother tried to help and comfort her. On Easter Sunday Ann was told that there was no hope. We went to nearby Westminster Cathedral and prayed. It was three o'clock. On our return to the hospital Ann was called to the ward. Leanne held up her hand to hold her mother's and died instantly and peacefully. It was as though she had been waiting for her.

Ann burst with grief, cursed the vicar and said she couldn't ever pray again.

By the time Ann's husband arrived Leanne was dead. They had been in hospital over a year. Ann's marriage, like many others I had witnessed in the mothers' unit, was crumbling.

After the funeral she left her husband and they sold up their home. Ann came back to the hospital to see us.

'You know, gran,' she said, addressing my mother, 'one minute I'm a wife and a mother, and the next I'm nothing.'

We understood.

Earnestly she continued. 'I can't really believe she's gone. Sometimes I think it's just a bad dream – that right now I can walk onto the ward and she'll be there. I'll lift her into my arms and she'll be soft and warm. You know, my man thought I would do something to myself, but I won't. I know Leanne is in a better place. I read somewhere that if you commit suicide, you don't go anywhere. I couldn't bear the thought of not being with Leanne. So, you see, she's giving me strength to go on, isn't she? Then the doctors told me that they learnt such a lot from Leanne's transplant which will help other children, so she didn't die for nothing, did she? There is some purpose behind it all, isn't there?'

I've asked myself the same question a thousand times.

Epilogue

I remember my joy when once I had a son. I had so many dreams of our future together. I wanted so much for him; to guide him, with love, through his illness to healthy manhood.

Those dreams were shattered when Anthony died on the evening of Sunday 21 October 1979 aged just seven years. Those were seven years of happiness and heartache during which we battled together for his health and freedom; seven years during which our special love-bond grew with the realisation of my privilege to be the mother of such a brave and beautiful son.

A gentle, sensitive boy, Anthony enjoyed music, poetry and painting. He loved to pick flowers and delighted in their variety of perfume, shape and colour. His favourite flower was the simple daisy. Did he realise, I wonder, how swiftly the daisy blooms and dies? To me it is a sad analogy of his own short life.

Few children can have generated such love and respect. He was adored by everyone who came to know him personally, indeed, by many thousands more who learned of his courage. Anthony created his own world-family who now grieve with me at his death.

Anthony also motivated a world-wide flow of prayer. It was always a great comfort, especially during our long periods of isolation and intense loneliness, to learn that in so many countries, those of different ethnic origin and religious belief gathered to pray for us.

I believe that Anthony represented much more than the struggle to establish a bone marrow transplant programme in Britain. He represented then and still represents now the rights of the individual in our society, especially those of children and their basic human right of a chance to lead a normal, healthy life.

The groundwork of our vital medical project is only possible due to the overwhelming support of the public and media. There is still much in this field of medicine that is still pioneer work. We have a long, hard road ahead but I look to the day when no child dies like my son, waiting for a donor to save him.

The Anthony Nolan Laboratories exist, the technicians are trained and working, the lifeline is strong and we are now full of hope for future generations.

Anthony was a symbol of hope. If his tragic death is to have any meaning, I implore everyone with children of their own and parents of the future to support Anthony's Memorial Appeal, to ensure that our vital medical project comes to fruition to give life to other children as a tribute to a truly remarkable little boy, Anthony Nolan.

Shirley Nolan
28 October 1979

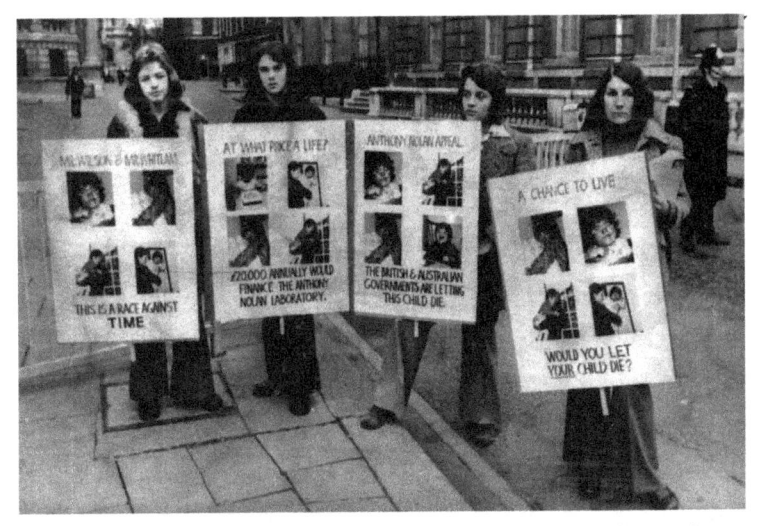

Shirley Nolan campaigning outside No.10 Downing Street, December 1974.

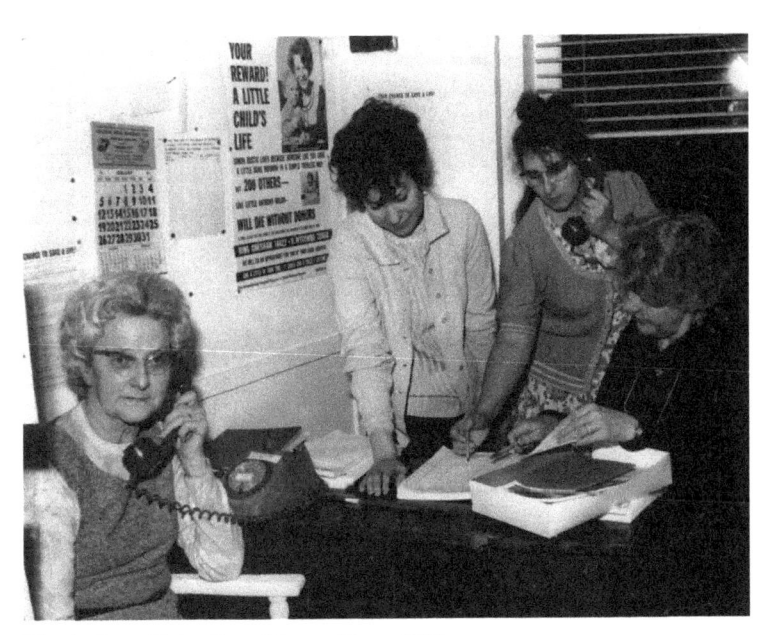

The Anthony Nolan Bone Marrow Trust, 1975.

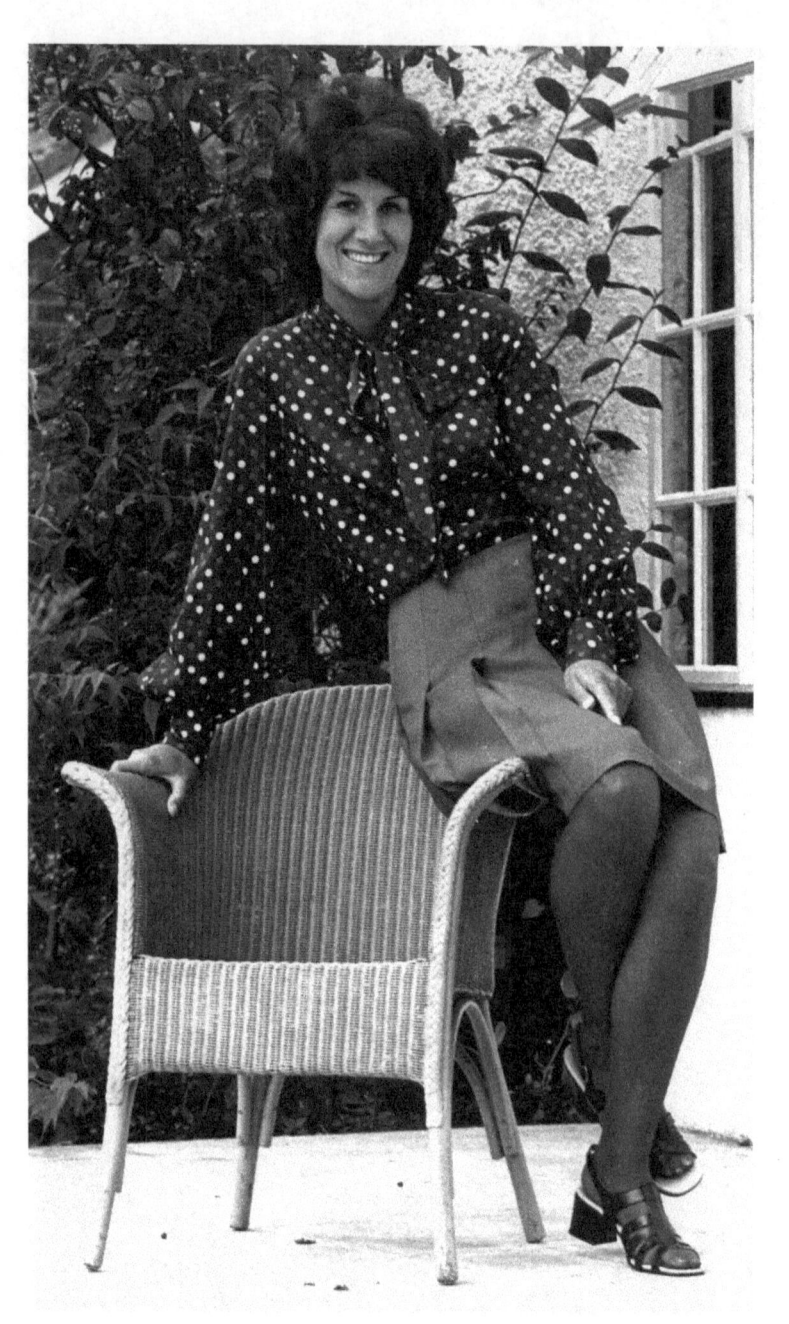

Shirley Nolan.

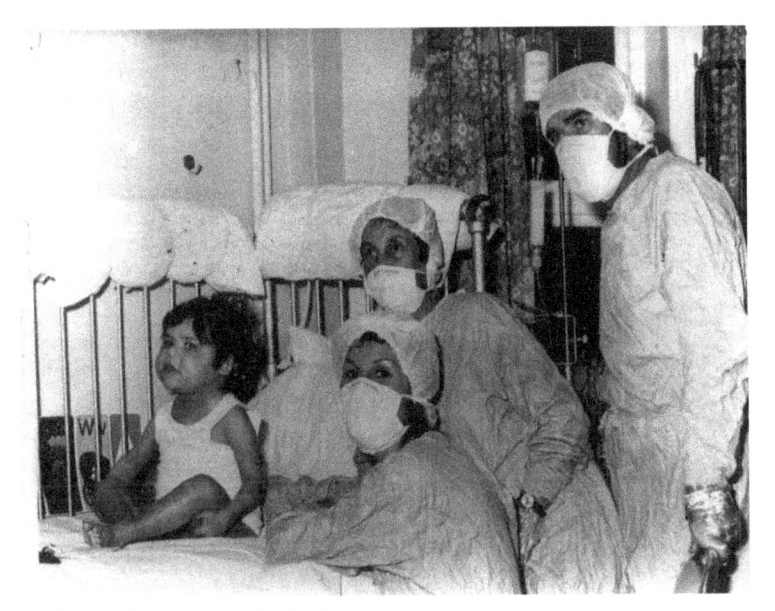

Anthony in hospital with his family.

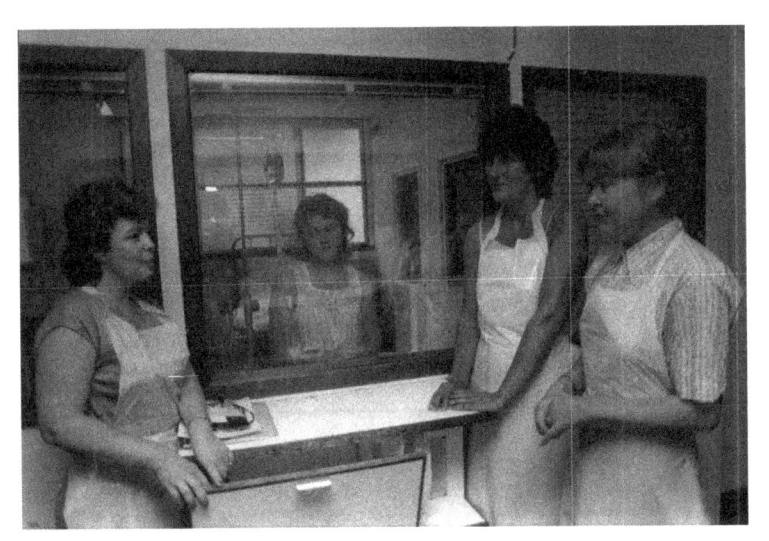

Shirley talking to nurses in hospital.

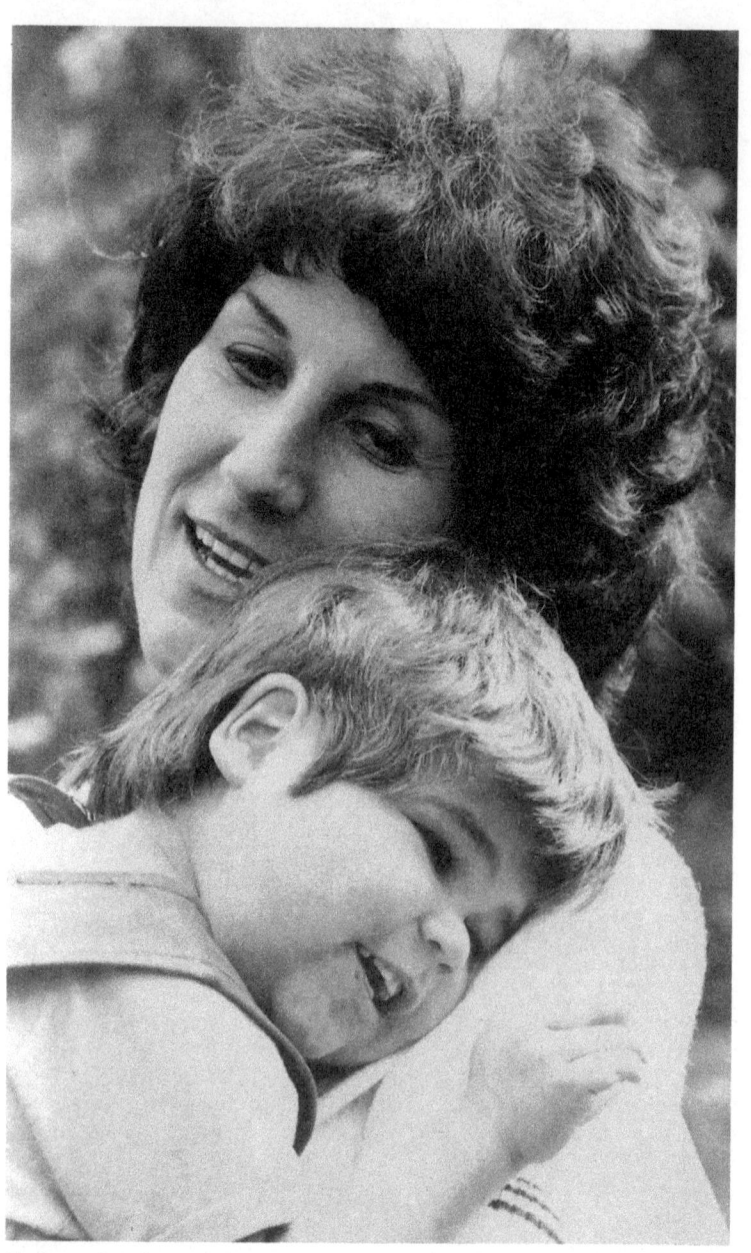

Shirley and Anthony Nolan.

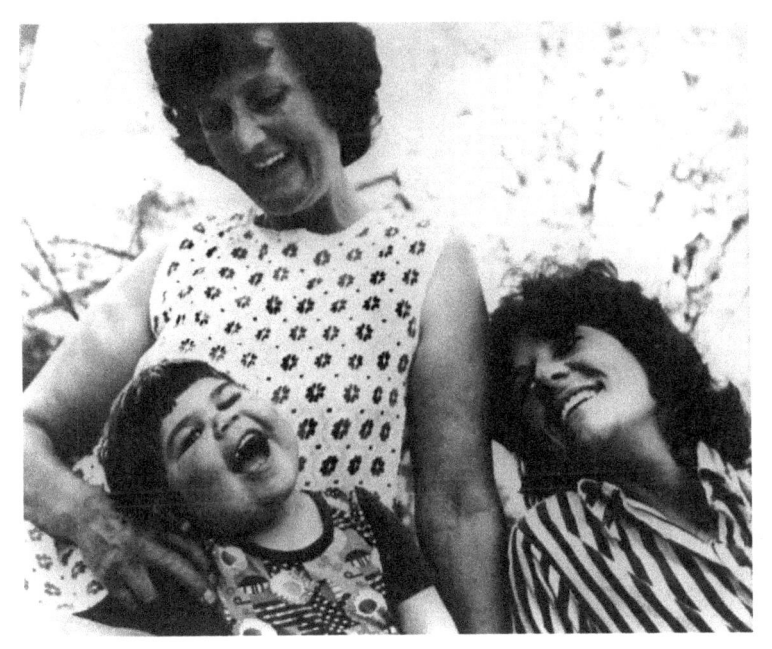

Shirley with her mother Rhoda and Anthony.

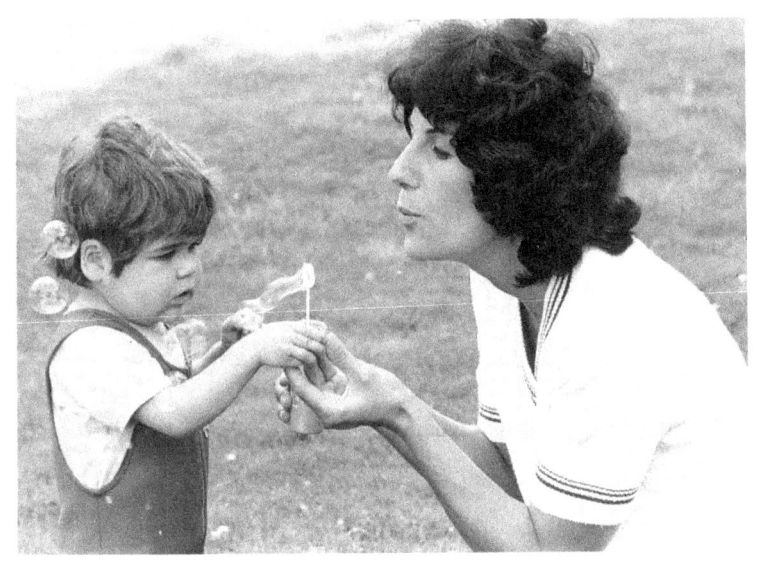

Shirley and Anthony Nolan.

Support Anthony Nolan Today

Since Shirley Nolan launched the world's first stem cell register in 1974, her son Anthony's story has given the hope of a lifesaving transplant to thousands of people with blood cancer or a blood disorder. It's a story about the power of a mother's love and a vision that has saved thousands of lives.

To mark the 50th anniversary of our charity, Anthony Nolan, we're celebrating Shirley's legacy and the incredible progress she brought to the way blood cancer and blood disorders are treated.

We are immensely proud to say that through our groundbreaking research, our lifesaving register, and our exceptional patient care, we save the lives of four people every single day. However, it is only thanks to the generosity of our amazing supporters that we can continue all of Anthony Nolan's work saving lives through stem cells.

Adding each new lifesaving stem cell donor onto our register costs £40. That cost includes recruiting a donor, plus collecting and analysing each new donor's sample to work out their tissue type. We then securely store the donor's tissue type on our register so we can search for them as a match for someone with blood cancer. Please do consider supporting Anthony Nolan with a financial gift of whatever you can afford.

You can donate online at: **www.anthonynolan.org**

With each new potential donor that we can add to the stem cell register, you could be helping to save a patient's life, ensuring that Shirley's legacy lives on.